John Ebnezar CBS | Handbooks in Orthopedics and Fractures

SERIES

Specific Orthopedic Problems

Orthopedic Problems of Forearm

John Ebnezar

- Holder of the **Guinness Book of World Records** for the most number of books written by an individual in a single year.
- Listed in the **India Book of Records** for the most number of books written by an individual.
- Recipient of the highest civilian awards of Karnataka, the **Rajyotsava Award 2010** and the **Kempegowda Award 2011**.
- Recipient of the **Best Citizen of India Award** by the International Publishing house.
- Former Vice-President, the Indian Orthopaedic Association
- President, Neuro-Spinal Surgeons Association of India (Karnataka)
- CEO, Parimala Health Care Services, A ISO 9001:2008 Hospital, Bilekahalli, Bannerghatta Road, Bangalore
- Ebnezar Orthopedic Center, Bilekahalli, Bannerghatta Road, Bangalore
- Dr John's Orthopedic Clinic, near Reliance Mart, Arakere, BG Road, Bangalore
- Chairman, the Physically Handicapped and Paraplegic Charitable Trust of Karnataka®
- Founder President, Geriatric Orthopedic Society
- Founder President, Orthopedic Authors Association and All India Medical Authors Association
- Chairman, Karnataka Orthopedic Academy®
- President, Bangalore Holistic Academy
- Chairman, Rakesh Cultural Academy
- President, Vaidya Kala Ranga, Bangalore
- Secretary, SK Educational Society®
- Former Senior Specialist, Victoria Hospital, Bangalore Medical College, Bangalore
- Former Assistant Professor in Orthopedics, Devaraj Urs Medical College, Kolar, Karnataka
- Postgraduate teacher, Bangalore Baptist Hospital, Airport Road, Bangalore

John Ebnezar CBS | Handbooks in
Orthopedics and Fractures

SERIES

Specific Orthopedic Problems

Orthopedic Problems of Forearm

John Ebnezar

MBBS, D'Ortho, DNB (Ortho), MNAMS (Ortho), PhD (Yoga)
Sports Medicine (Australia), INOR Fellow (UK), DAc, DMT

Consulting Orthopedic and Spine Surgeon,
Holistic Orthopedic Expert, and Sports Specialist
Bangalore

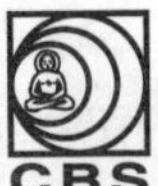

CBS Publishers & Distributors Pvt Ltd
New Delhi • Bengaluru • Pune • Kochi • Chennai

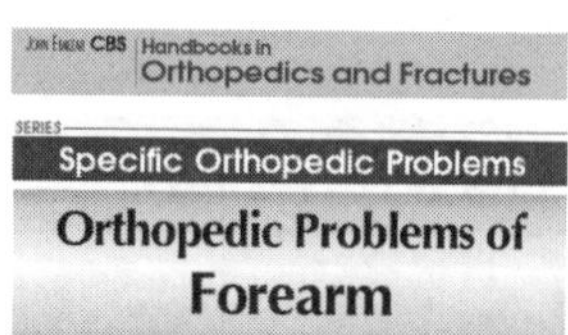

> *Disclaimer*
> Science and technology are constantly changing fields. New research and experience broaden the scope of information and knowledge. The author has tried his best in giving information available to him while preparing the material for this book. Although, all efforts have been made to ensure optimum accuracy of the material, yet it is quite possible some errors might have been left uncorrected. The publisher, printer and author will not be held responsible for any inadvertent errors or inaccuracies.

ISBN: 978-81-239-2123-5

First Edition: 2012

Published by Satish Kumar Jain and produced by Vinod K. Jain for
CBS Publishers & Distributors Pvt Ltd
4819/XI Prahlad Street, 24 Ansari Road, Daryaganj
New Delhi 110 002, India.
Ph: 23289259, 23266861, 23266867
Fax: 011-23243014
Website: www.cbspd.com
e-mail: delhi@cbspd.com
cbspubs@airtelmail.in.

Branches

- Bengaluru: Seema House 2975, 17th Cross, K.R. Road, Banasankari 2nd Stage, Bengaluru 560 070, Karnataka
  Ph: +91-80-26771678/79 Fax: +91-80-26771680 e-mail: bangalore@cbspd.com
- Pune: Bhuruk Prestige, Sr. No. 52/12/2+1+3/2 Narhe, Haveli (Near Katraj-Dehu Road Bypass), Pune 411 051, Maharashtra
  Ph: 020-64704058, 64704059, 32392277 Fax: +91-020-24300160 e-mail: pune@cbspd.com
- Kochi: 36/14 Kalluvilakam, Lissie Hospital Road, Kochi 682 018, Kerala
  Ph: +91-484-4059061-65 Fax: +91-484-4059065 e-mail: cochin@cbspd.com
- Chennai: 20, West Park Road, Shenoy Nagar, Chennai 600 030, Tamil Nadu
  Ph: +91-44-26260666, 26208620 Fax: +91-44-45530020 email: chennai@cbspd.com

Printed at Magic International, Greater Noida (UP)

to

---

my mother
(late) Sampath Kumari
who taught me that life is more than self and
there is more joy in giving and sharing than taking

my wife
Dr Parimala

my lovely children
Rakesh and Priyanka
who are an epitome of love, sacrifice, encouragement
and inspiration

all my teachers
who made me what I am today

all my students
past and present

and

all my patients

Dr John Ebnezar

is a legendary name as a prolific orthopedic writer. No other orthopedic surgeon in the world has come anywhere close to him in the number of books he has written in his field. He is the first orthopedic surgeon in the world to be listed in the **Guinness Book of World Records** for the most number of books written by an individual in a single year. For the same feat his name has been listed in the **India Book of Records.** This book, like all his previous books, carries his flavor of simple and lucid writing, excellent language, beautiful illustrations and excellent presentation of the topics. This book is a part of the 100^{+} book series he has brought out in a single calendar year of 2012 on a wide array of orthopedic problems of public health importance. No other individual in the world has brought out these many books in one year and this is a world record attempt. With these books he aims to educate the reader and the public about these common orthopedic problems.

All his books have been accepted very well and he has a great fan following all over the world. He has been bestowed with as many as 32 international, national and state awards including Karnataka state's highest civilian award the **Rajyotsava Award 2010** and the **Kempegowda Award 2011,** apart from the **Best Citizen of India Award** given by the International Publishing House. He is the pioneer in holistic orthopedics and is credited for discovering a new method of treatment for the common orthopedic problems and has done PhD in arthritis from the world famous S-VYASA University, Bangalore. He is currently president of the Neuro-Spinal Surgeons Association of India (Karnataka), the former Vice-President of the Indian Orthopedic Association, and is the founder president of various orthopedic bodies.

Preface

This book is a part of the 100^+ book series

JOHN EBNEZAR CBS Handbooks in Orthopedics and Fractures

which deals with the orthopedic problems of public health importance. The purpose of these books is to educate and create awareness among the readers about various problems associated with orthopedics. Through this way the readers get to know all about various orthopedic problems directly from a specialist. This will help a reader immensely in getting the right knowledge as most of them depend on the internet and magazines which distort and misrepresent various pieces of information concerning health topics, leaving the readers confused and worse still improperly educated. This may harm more than helping them find solutions to their problems. The purpose of these books, therefore, is to educate the readers right in their quest for knowledge on the common health and associated problems.

The 100^+ book series has been brought out in a single calendar year.

Orthopedic problems encountered by the people all over the world can be classified into two broad categories, traumatic and non-traumatic conditions. These problems are on the rise thanks to the increased instances of RTA's, natural calamaties, and rise in orthopedic lifestyle problems. This book deals with all the orthopedic problems of the forearm, both traumatic and non-traumatic, some of which are common and some not so common. They come with their own unique set of problems. This is the first ever book which exclusively deals with specific orthopedic problems of the forearm, and I have made an attempt to bring all the important basic aspects about these conditions in one book, so that the reader gets to know about them.

Highlights of this book

- Simple and lucid language
- Good illustrations
- Good Clinical photograph wherever necessary

- Relevant X-rays
- Short summaries
- Anecdotes

This book has ubiquitous utility and usage and can be useful to the orthopedic surgeons, postgraduate students in orthopedics, undergraduate medical students, doctors from all disciplines of medicine, physiotherapists, therapists practising alternative systems of medicine, rehabilitation specialists, and most importantly the common people. It is particularly useful to those unsung heroes who work in remote areas with minimum infrastructure. They can use this book as a ready-reckoner. Seldom will you find a book that covers such a wide spectrum of readers.

Knowing about the all the orthopedic problems affecting your forearm, creates an awareness about these conditions and helps one to understand them better and take the necessary preventive steps in preventing them from happening at the first place and if unfortunately, if one is a victim of these conditions, it helps them to know and understand everything about the cause, presentation, investigations and treatment your doctor recommends for them.

Constructive criticism and useful suggestions are invited to make the book more effective in its forthcoming editions.

John Ebnezar

Acknowledgments

This volume is a part of the 100^{+} book series brought out in a single calendar year. This was a huge and mammoth task attempted first time ever by an author and a publisher in the world. Such an herculean effort could not have been possible without the active involvement of those concerned in CBS Publishers & Distributors. I thank Mr Satish K Jain, Managing Director of CBS P&D, for agreeing to be a part of this world-record feat in bringing out this book in the Series. My special thanks to Mr YN Arjuna who showed special interest in this work and channelized his entire energy into this improbable feat. My special thanks to Mrs Ritu Chawla and her entire dedicated team who have toiled day and night to make this dream a reality. I thank members of the entire editorial–production team of CBS P&D who have worked hard behind the scenes to bring out this book.

My special thanks to Dr Yogitha for actively helping me in the compilation of all the books. I also thank all the staff members of my hospital who have helped me at various levels during the making of this book.

John Ebnezar

Contents

John Ebnezar **CBS** | Handbooks in
Orthopedics and Fractures

TITLES IN THE SERIES

I Orthopedic Trauma

General Fractures

1 General Principles of Fractures and Dislocations
2 Fracture Treatment Methods
3 Fractures and their Complications
4 Atypical Fractures

Injuries of Upper Limb

5 Injuries of Shoulder
6 Injuries of Arm
7 Injuries of Elbow
8 Injuries of Forearm
9 Injuries of Wrist and Hand
10 Injuries of Distal Forearm and Wrist
11 Injuries of Hand
12 Injuries of Upper Limb

Injuries of Lower Limb

13 Injuries of Hip
14 Injuries of Femur
15 Injuries of Knee
16 Injuries of Knee and Leg
17 Injuries of Ankle and Leg
18 Injuries of Foot and Ankle
19 Injuries of Lower Limb

Injuries of Axial Skeleton

20 Injuries of Pelvis and Hip
21 Injuries of Spine
22 Injuries of Pelvis and Spine

23 Sports Injuries Volume I
24 Sports Injuries Volume II
25 Soft Tissue Problems in Orthopedics
26 Geriatric Trauma
27 Pediatric Trauma

II Orthopedic Disease

28 Congenital Orthopedic Problems
29 Developmental Orthopedic Problems

III Specific Orthopedic Problems

IV Regional Orthopedic Problems

V Orthopedic Injuries and Surgeries

VI Practical Examination

VII Orthopedic Problems of Different Ages

VIII Common Orthopedic Problems

IX Yoga Therapy in Common Orthopedic Problems

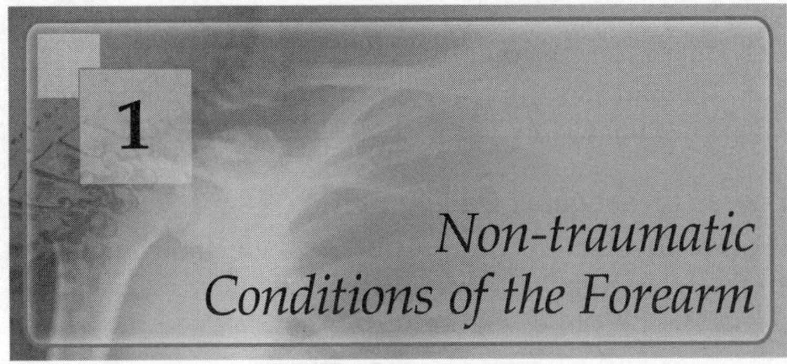

1 Non-traumatic Conditions of the Forearm

This chapter deals with important non-traumatic conditions of the forearm.

CONGENITAL FOREARM CONDITIONS

CONGENITAL RADIOULNAR SYNOSTOSIS

In the normal person, forearm bones called the radius and ulna lie separately and are united above and below by two joints. I call this an unholy alliance of radius and ulna for their union causes unmitigated hardship to the sufferer.

What are the Salient features?

- Involves proximal ends of radius and ulna.
- Bones fix the forearm in pronation.
- Bilateral.
- Familial tendency.

Classification (For medical readers)

Two types are described, Type I and Type II.

How does the patient present? Clinical Features

The patient presents with

- Deformity of the upper forearm and
- The forearm could be fixed in mid-pronation.
- There is no pronation and supination movements of the forearm.

- Elbow flexion could remain unaffected.
- The patient complains of difficulty in carrying out his day-to-day activities with the affected forearm.

How to Investigate? Radiograph

Plain X-ray of the forearm including both elbow and wrist joints are essential to diagnose this condition (Fig. 1.1).

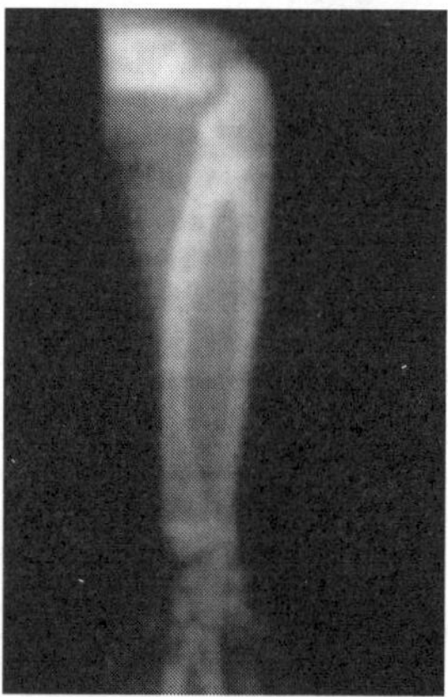

Fig. 1.1: Radiograph showing congenital radioulnar synostosis

Reasons for difficulty in treatment

- Fascial tissues are short.
- Interosseous membrane is narrow.
- Supinator muscle is abnormal or absent.

How to manage this condition? Treatment

Treatment is limited to osteotomy, to place the forearm in midprone position for better function.

Attempts to overcome the synostosis and give rotatory function to the forearm are doomed to failure because of the lack of properly functioning muscles. Fortunately, most patients are not disabled enough to justify an extensive operation.

MADELUNG'S DEFORMITY

It is an abnormality of the *palmar ulnar part of the distal radial epiphysis* in which progressive ulnar and volar tilt develops at the distal radial articular surface, resulting in dorsal subluxation of the distal ulna.

First described by Malgaigne in 1855 and later by Madelung in 1878.

Though congenital, it is not obvious until late childhood and adolescence. It is a rare condition, incidence being only 1.7 percent.

What are the Causes?

The causes could be autosomal dominant, dysplasic (diaphysial aclasis), genetic or idiopathic.

Acquired deformities distinguished by lack of appropriate physical findings, unilateral, less severe carpal deformities, and history of repetitive injury or stress.

How does the patient present? Clinical Features

Madelung's deformity consists of:

- Volar subluxation of hand.
- Prominence of distal ulna.
- Volar and ulnar angulation of distal radius (Fig. 1.2).

Other Features

This condition is

- Commonly bilateral

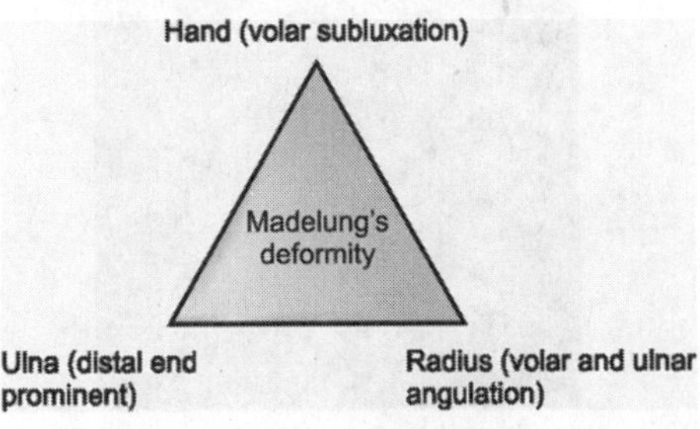

Fig. 1.2: Madelung's deformity

- Girls are more affected.
- There is a positive family history.
- The deformity manifests in late childhood and adolescents with restricted wrist motion and minimal pain.
- As growth occurs, deformity worsens and the forearm is short.

How to detect this problem? Plain X-rays are the investigation of choice

Radiographic abnormalities are seen in radius, ulna and carpal bones.

- Radius is curved with its convexity dorsal and radial.
- Distal radial epiphysis is triangular because of the failure of the growth in the ulnar and volar aspects of the epiphysis. Early closure of these aspects of epiphysis is frequent.
- Ulna is subluxated dorsally, its head is enlarged and the overall length of ulna is decreased. Carpus appears to have subluxated ulnaward and palmarwards into the distal radioulnar joint.
- Carpus appears wedge-shaped with its apex proximal (Fig. 1.3).

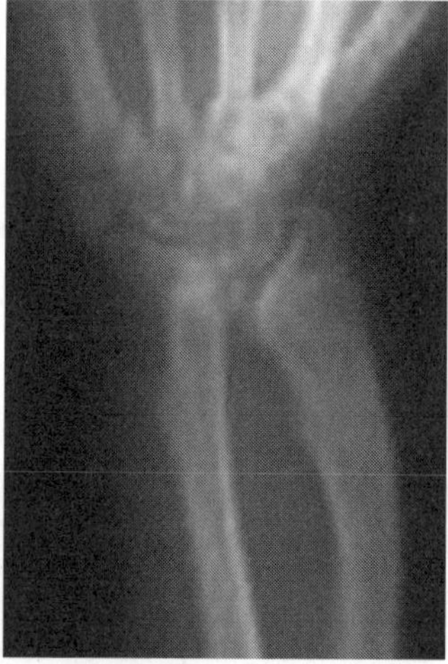

Fig. 1.3: Radiograph of Madelung's deformity

How to manage this problem? Treatment

Conservative Treatment

Children with Madelung's deformity have minimal pain and excellent function. Hence, conservative treatment is given initially.

Surgery

Surgery is considered for severe deformity or persistent pain. In skeletally immature patients, distal radial osteotomy with ulnar shortening is (Milch resection) preferred. In skeletally mature patients, osteotomy and Darrach's procedure are done. Deformity may recur after either procedure and range of motion of forearm usually does not improve after surgery.

CONGENITAL ABSENCE OF RADIUS (RADIAL CLUBHAND)

Failure of the formation of the parts along the preaxial or radial borders of the upper extremity, deficient or absent thenar muscles, short or absent thumb, short or absent radius.

Quick facts

- One in one lakh birth.
- Incidence—4.7 percent.
- Bilateral in 50 percent of cases.
- Sexes equal.
- Right side more common.
- Complete absence more common than partial absence.
- Cause unknown/thalidomide/genetic.

Heikel's Classification (For medical readers only)

Type I : Short distal radius.
Type II : Hypoplastic radius.
Type III : Partial absence of radius.
Type IV : Total absence of radius (most common).

How does the patient present? Clinical Features

The patient presents with

- Deformity of the forearm and wrist.
- The forearm appears short and small and the deformity of the forearm, wrist and hand are quite grotesque (Fig.1.4A).
- The forearm and hand functions are severely affected.
- The patient complains of difficulty in carrying out his day-to-day activities with the affected forearm.

Radiograph

Plain X-ray of the forearm including both elbow and wrist joints are essential to diagnose this condition (Fig. 1.4B).

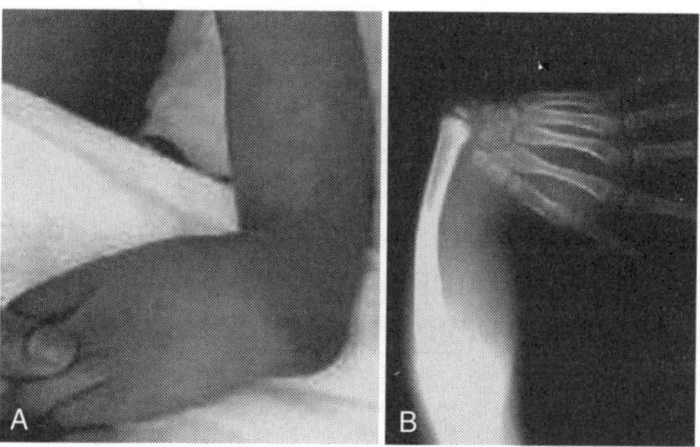

Figs 1.4A and B: (A) Radial clubhand (Clinical photo), (B) Radiograph of radial clubhand

How to manage? Treatment

After birth, the deformity is corrected passively and splinted with a short arm plastic splint. Surgical correction, i.e. centralization of hands is usually done at 3–6 months. Pollicization is done at 9–12 months.

CONGENITAL DISLOCATION OF RADIUS

This is uncommon and is often confused with Monteggia's fractures.

How does the patient present? Clinical Features

- A prominent head of the radius is felt in the upper forearm.
- Forearm function of supination and pronation are affected but the elbow movements remain normal.
- Due to long standing dislocation there could be pain and features of secondary OA of the superoradioulnar joint.

Radiology

Plain X-ray of the elbow and entire forearm is advised to detect this lesion with reasonable accuracy (Fig. 1.5).

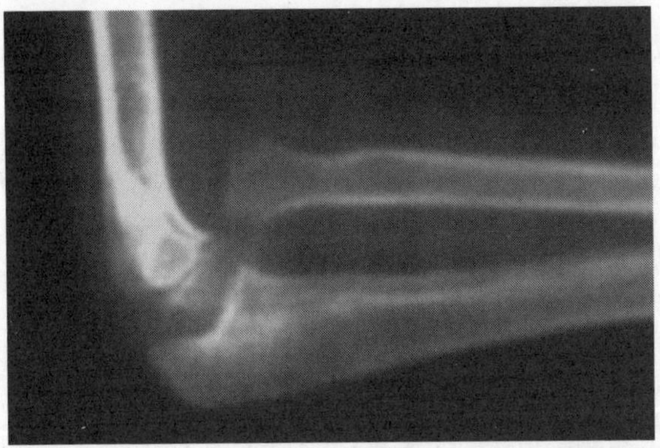

Fig. 1.5: Radiograph showing congenital dislocation of radius

How to manage? Treatment

This is treated surgically and consists of excision of the head of radius after skeletal maturity.

REGIONAL DISORDERS OF FOREARM

TENNIS ELBOW

I am sure everyone is fascinated by tennis. We may not get a place under the sun with Roger Federer, Nadal, Pete Sampras, Leander Paes, Sania Mirza and others, but certainly, we may get an appointment with an orthopedic surgeon for a problem common in them, that too without playing tennis! Yes, the obvious reference is towards *tennis elbow.*

> *Note:* Sachin Tendulkar should be credited for popularizing and creating lots of awareness and controversies about tennis elbow at least in our country!

History

It was first described from the *Writer's cramps* by Range in 1873. It was Madris who called it as "tennis elbow" shortly thereafter.

Definition

Tennis elbow syndrome encompasses lateral, medial and posterior elbow symptoms. The one commonly encountered is the lateral tennis elbow which is known as the ***classical tennis elbow*** and is the *pain and tenderness on the lateral side of the elbow,* some well-defined and some vague, that results from repetitive stress.

Tennis elbow	
Classical tennis elbow	*Other varieties*
• It is the lateral tennis elbow	• Medial tennis elbow *(Golfer's elbow)* • Posterior tennis elbow around the margins of the olecranon process

Vital points

Location of pain in tennis elbow

- Lateral epicondyle (75%)
- Lateral muscle mass (17%)
- Medial epicondyle (10%)
- Posterior (8%).

Lateral Tennis Elbow

It is a lesion affecting the tendinous origin of common wrist extensors (Fig. 1.6). It is more common in men than women are and is believed to be a degenerative disorder.

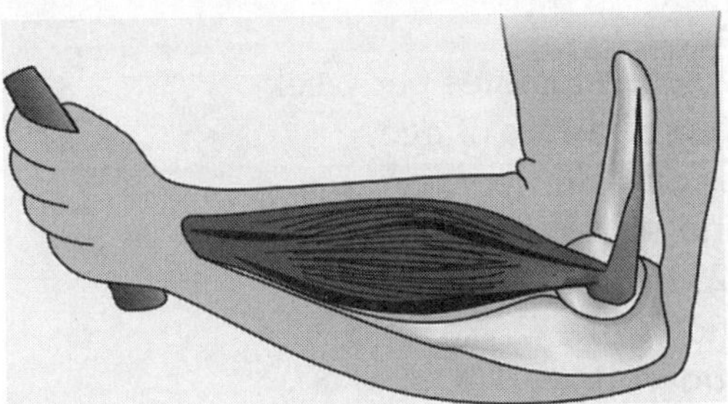

Fig. 1.6: Repetitive stress at common extensor origin in tennis players

Causes

Epicondylitis: This is due to single or multiple tears in the common extensor origin, periostitis, angiofibroblastic proliferation of extensor carpi radialis brevis (ECRB), etc.

Inflammation of adventitious bursa: Between the common extensor origin and radio humeral joint.

Calcified deposits: Within the common extensor tendon.

Painful annular ligament: It is due to hypertrophy of synovial fringe between the radial head and the capitulum's.

Pain of neurological origin, e.g. cervical spine affection, radial nerve entrapment, etc.

Mystifying fact

ECRB is the most commonly involved structure in lateral epicondylitis.

Seen in

- All levels of tennis players.
- In world class players "SERVE" appears to be the cause.
- In less than world class players "backhand stroke".
- Seen in other sports also.
- May be occupational, etc.
- More common in the dominated arm.

Causes in tennis players: More than one-third tennis players all over the world are affected with this problem over 35 years of age.

- Novice
- Playing several games per week
- More than 35 years of age
- Equal sex incidence
- Backhand stroke (38%)
- Serve (25%)
- Forehand stroke (23%)
- Backhand volley (7%)
- Overhead smash (4%)
- Forehand volley (3%)

Contributing factors

- Little playing experience.
- Consistent missing of "*sweet spot*" while hitting.
- Poor stroke techniques: Use of arm instead of body.
- Poor power or flexibility.
- Heavy stiff racket, large handle size, too tight racket stringing.
- Heavy duty wet balls.
- Playing surface—balls bounce quicker off the cement court.

Did you know?

Though called tennis elbow, it is more common in non-tennis players (95%). Causes can be:

- Throwing sports
- Swimming
- Carpentry, plumbing, textile workers
- Housewives

However, up to 50 percent of tennis players suffer from this problem at some time in their sporting career.

Pathophysiology and Related Symptoms

Stage I: There is acute inflammation but no angioblastic invasion. *The patient complains of pain during activity.*

Stage II: This is the stage of chronic inflammation. There is some angioblastic invasion. *The patient complains of pain both during activity and at rest.*

Stage III: Chronic inflammation with extensive angioblastic invasion. *The patient complains pain at rest, night pains, and pain during daily activities.*

Etiology

Problems in tennis players: More than one-third tennis players all over the world are affected with this problem over 35 years of age are obviously due to faculty playing techniques.

Nontennis players: Ironically tennis elbow is more common is nontennis players. This unfortunate group is comprised of housewives, carpenters, miners, drill workers, etc. India's Cricketing Legend Sachin Tendulkar and Sreesanth have made tennis elbow very popular across the country and the world.

Indian housewives: This is the third largest group suffering from this condition. The household chores like washing, brooming, cooking, etc. require repeated extension of the elbow leading to the development of this condition.

Computer related injuries: This is emerging as the recent epidemic among computer professionals across the globe due to repetitive stress while using laptops, mouse, etc.

Clinical Features

Patient complains of pain on the outer aspect of the elbow and has difficulty in gripping objects and lifting them. Sportspersons will have difficulty in extending the elbow. The following are some of the useful clinical tests.

Clinical Tests

Local tenderness on the outside of the elbow at the common extensor origin with aching pain in the back of the forearm (Fig. 1.7).

Cozen's test: Painful resisted extension of the wrist with elbow in full extension elicits pain at the lateral elbow (Fig. 1.8).

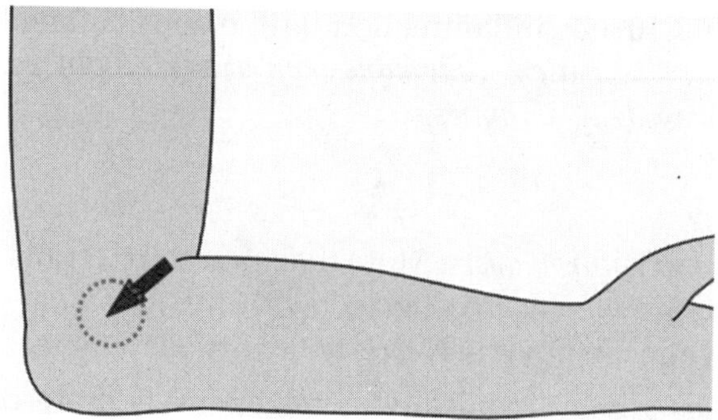

Fig. 1.7: Arrow showing site of tenderness in tennis elbow

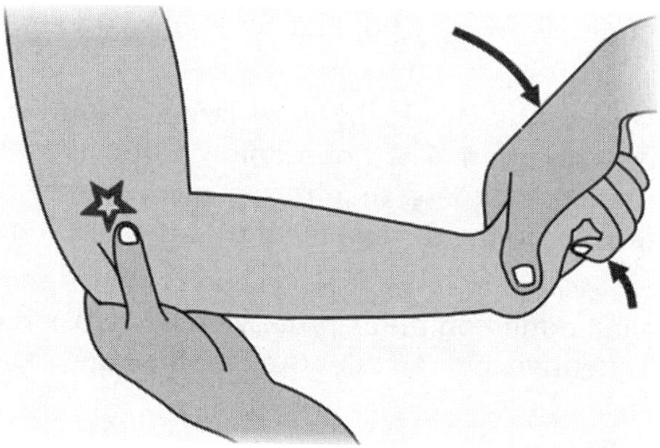

Fig. 1.8: Method of performing the Cozen's test

Elbow held in extension, passive wrist flexion and pronation produces pain.

Maudsley's test: Resisted extension of the middle finger (Remember the letter 'M') elicits pain at the lateral epicondyle due to disease in the extensor digitorum communis.

Radiograph for Tennis Elbow

The AP, lateral and radiocapitellar views are the recommended views. In most cases, it is normal. However, in 16 percent of the cases, a faint calcification along the lateral epicondyle can be detected.

Treatment

Conservative Management

It consists of rest and physiotherapy. In tennis players exercises, light racket, smaller grip, elbow strap, etc. are helpful (Fig. 1.9). Injection of local anesthetic and steroid are useful in 40 percent of cases.

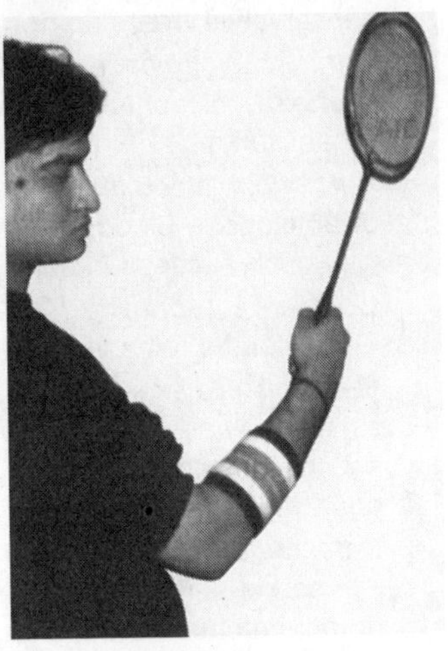

Fig. 1.9: Elbow supports to be used in tennis elbow

Mill's Maneuver

This is the final option before surgery. About 10 percent of the cases do not respond to conservative treatment. In them, a forceful extension of a fully flexed and pronated forearm after injection may be attempted.

Surgical Management

Indications

- Severe pain for 6 weeks at least.
- Marked and localized tenderness over lateral epicondyle.
- Failure to respond to restricted activity or immobilization for at least 2 weeks.

Surgical Methods

- Percutaneous release of epicondylar muscles.
- Bosworth technique of excision of the proximal portion of the annular ligament, release of the origin of the extensor muscles, excision of the bursa and excision of synovial fringes.

What is new in the treatment of Tennis and Golfer's elbow?

- *The use of extracorporeal shock wave therapy (ESWT):* About 2,000 shock waves of 0.04–0.12 nj/mm^2, three times at monthly intervals for 6 months are found to be effective in cases with failed conservative treatment for at least 6 months.
- *Arthroscopic release:* Of ECRB with failed conservative treatment for nearly 6 months. It is minimally invasive and helps in early rehabilitation.
- *Autologous blood injections:* In refractory cases, injections of 2 ml of autologous blood and 0.5 percent bupivicaine has been tried with good success in some centers.
- *Counterforce bracing (called the tennis elbow or forearm band):* These forces release the forces in the ECRB region.
- *Rehabilitative exercises:* These are wrist flexion, extension, forearm supination and pronation, wrist radial and ulnar deviations at three sets of ten repetitions everyday for 2–6 months is known to give good results.
- *Ultrasound-guided percutaneous needle therapy:* This consists of ultrasound-guided corticosteroid injection and needle debridement of the structures around lateral epicondyle.

Indications: In small tears, not responding to conservative therapy and if too small for surgery.

Advantages

- Minimally invasive procedure.
- Restoration of function is rapid.
- The option of surgery is still open.

In expert's hands, it has a success rate of 65 percent.

Quick facts

Significant relief of symptoms in tennis elbow:

• Changing tennis strokes	92 percent
• Stretching exercises	84 percent
• Use of splints	83 percent
• NSAIDs/steroid	85 percent
• Physiotherapy	50–75 percent
• Rest more than 1 month	72 percent

GOLFER'S ELBOW

(Syn: Epitrochleitis, Medial tennis elbow)

Did you know?
Golfer's elbow is also called Swimmer's elbow.

Definition

It is a tendinopathy of the insertion of the epitrochlear muscles [flexors of the fingers of the hand flexor carpi radialis (FCR) and pronators].

Epitrochleitis is very similar to lateral epicondylitis (tennis elbow) but occurs on the medial side of the elbow, where the pronator teres and the flexors of the wrist and fingers originate. Tensing of these muscles by resisted wrist and finger flexion in pronation will provoke the pain (Fig. 1.10).

Tenderness is often less well localized than in tennis elbow.

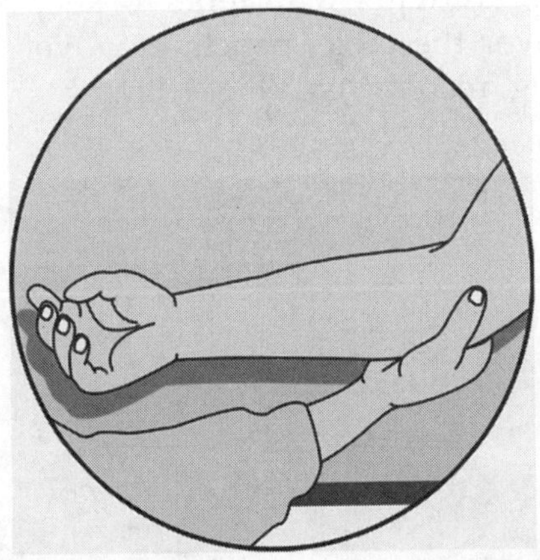

Fig. 1.10: Method of eliciting tenderness in golfer's elbow

Do you know?
Tennis elbow is nine times more common than golfer's elbow.

Treatment

It is the same as for tennis elbow, but the treatment is even less satisfactory.

Lesser-known but interesting elbow conditions

You know about tennis and golfer's elbow, but do you know about:

Boxer's elbow: This is also called as hyperextension overload syndrome or olecranon impingement syndrome and is due to the repetitive valgus hyperextension by a boxer during jabbing.

Little leagues elbow: This is a medial epicondyle avulsion fracture. It is seen commonly in children and adolescents involved in throwing sports.

OLECRANON BURSITIS (Student's Elbow) (Sign: Miner's elbow or Draughtsman elbow)

This is a chronic inflammation of the olecranon bursa. It may be the result of repetitive minor injuries or irritation, microcrystalline deposition. Infection occurs due to chronic friction as in students who tend to keep their elbows repeatedly over the table, bench, etc. over long periods during writing, reading, etc. (Fig. 1.11).

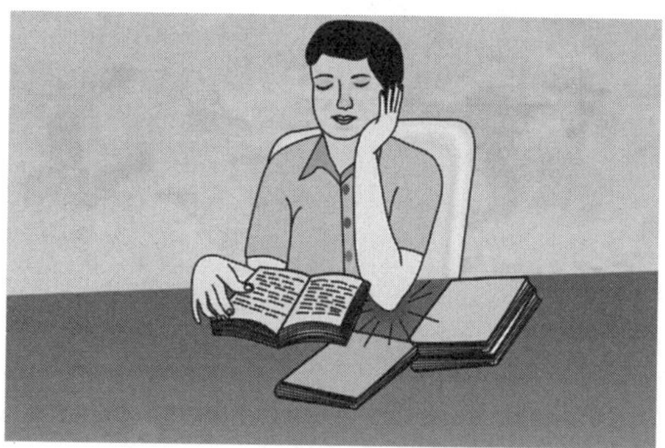

Fig. 1.11: Are you guilty of reading like this? Well you could develop student's elbow!

Clinical Features

It usually manifests as a swelling over the tip of the olecranon (Fig. 1.12). There may be pain, if there is inflammation. Inspection or palpation usually easily detects it (Fig. 1.13).

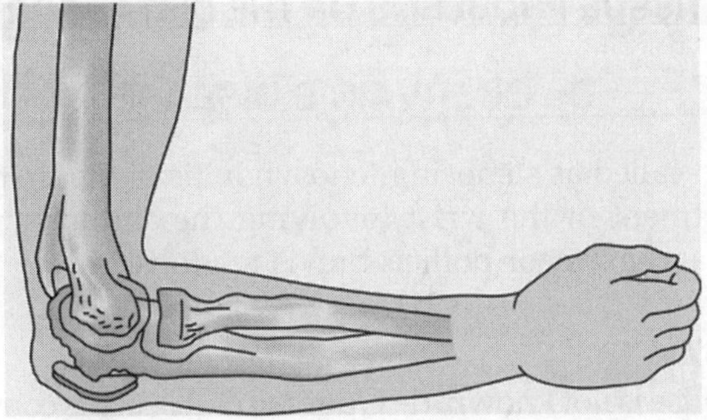

Fig. 1.12: Olecranon bursa

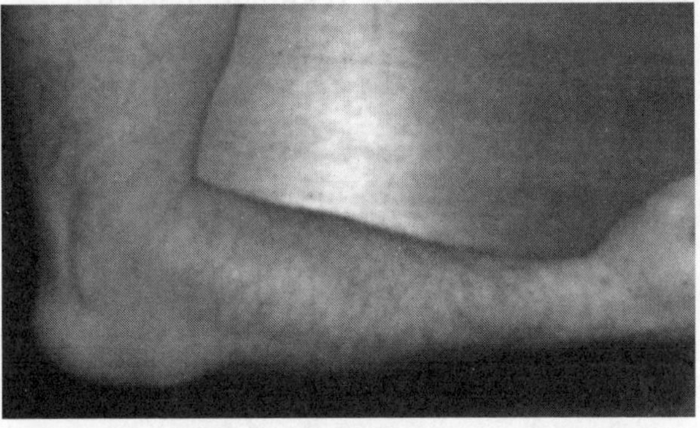

Fig. 1.13: Clinical picture of olecranon bursitis

Investigations

Aspiration and culture of the bursal fluid is necessary in order to exclude the possibility of an infectious etiology.

Treatment

Treatment is essentially conservative and consists of NSAIDs, local steroids, etc. Surgical excision is done in chronic cases. Microcrystalline-induced bursitis has a good prognosis and the symptoms usually resolve after a few days, whether treated or not. However, bursitis due to repeated minor irritation is more difficult to treat.

SOFT TISSUE PROBLEMS OF THE DISTAL FOREARM

De QUERVAIN'S DISEASE

It is also called as stenosing tenosynovitis of the first dorsal compartment of the wrist involving the abductor pollicis longus and extensor pollicis brevis tendons.

Etiology

Exact cause is not known. de Quervain's disease is commonly seen in women between 30 and 50 years of age, and may be due to repeated overuse of the wrist (Fig. 1.14). Trigger finger is common in conditions like rheumatoid arthritis.

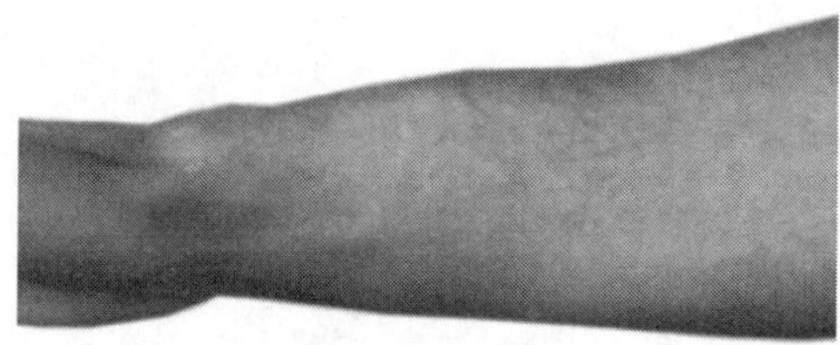

Fig. 1.14: Clinical photograph of de Quervain's disease

Clinical Features

Pain and limitation of the movements of the involved tendons are the presenting features. In this, the common sheath of abductor pollicis longus and extensor pollicis brevis tendons at the wrist are involved. Tenderness can be elicited by sudden ulnar deviation of the flexed hand [Finkelstein's test—with the thumb tucked inside the palm (Fig. 1.15)].

Pitfalls

Do you know that Finkelstein's test is not pathognomonic of de Quervain's disease? It is also positive in:

- First carpomatacarpal arthritis.
- Warrenberg's syndrome.
- Arthritis of radiocarpal and intercarpal joints.

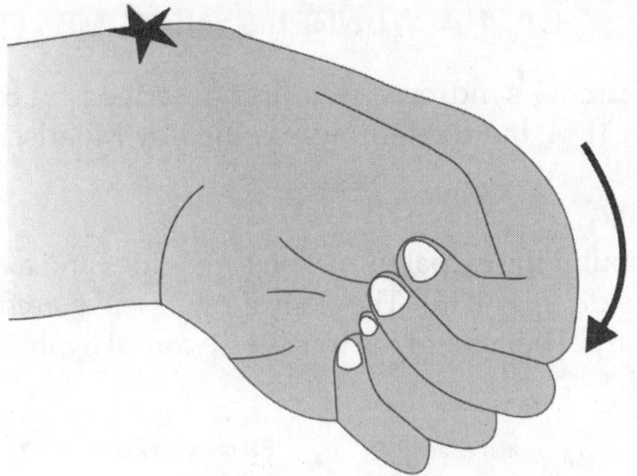

Fig. 1.15: Finkelstein's test

> **Interesting facts**
>
> Do you know about intersection syndrome? Well, it is tenosynovitis of the II dorsal compartment.

Treatment

Conservative Methods

This treatment consists of rest, NSAIDs, local infiltration of hydrocortisone, wrist immobilization, etc.

Surgery

Division of the appropriate retinaculum if the above measures fail.

> **Mystifying facts**
>
> **Do you know the reasons for failure of conservative treatment in de Quervain's disease?**
>
> - Anomalous tendons.
> - Multiple slips of abductor pollicis longus tendon.
> - Multiple subcompartments within the first wrist compartment. This is seen in 75 percent of the cases.

CARPAL TUNNEL SYNDROME

Carpal tunnel syndrome was first described by Sir James Paget in 1854, but the term was coined by Moerisch.

Anatomy

Bones bound the carpal tunnel on three sides and a ligament on one side (Fig. 1.16). The floor is an osseous arch formed by the carpal bones and the transverse carpal ligament forms the roof.

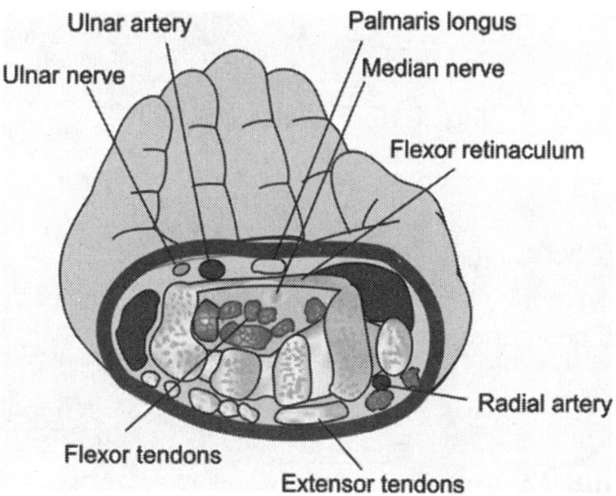

Fig. 1.16: Anatomy of the carpal tunnel

Contents

Tendons of flexor digitorum superficialis and profundus in a common sheath, tendon of flexor pollicis longus in an independent sheath and the median nerve (Fig. 1.17).

Synovitis of the above tendons can generate pressure on the nerve.

Know that 9 tendons and 1 nerve pass through the carpal tunnel.

Causes

General

Inflammatory—e.g. rheumatoid arthritis.

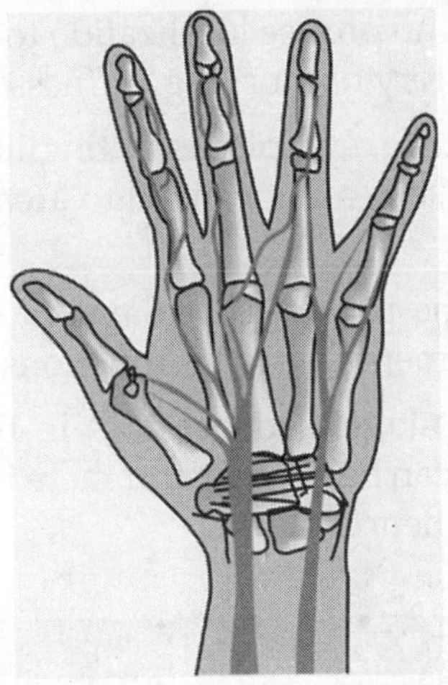

Fig. 1.17: Median nerve coursing through the carpal tunnel

Endocrine—hypothyroidism, diabetes mellitus, menopause, pregnancy, etc. are some of the important endocrine causes.
Metabolic cause—gout.

Local

These cause crowding of the space. Malunited Colles' fracture, ganglion in the carpal region, osteoarthritis of the carpal bones, and wrist contusion, hematoma, etc. are some of the important local causes.

> **Remember**
> Mnemonic PRAGMATIC for causes of carpal tunnel syndrome [(*P*—Pregnancy, *R*—Rheumatoid arthritis, *A*—Arthritis degenerative, *G*—Growth hormone abnormalities (acromegaly), *M*—Metabolic (gout, diabetes myxoedema, etc.), *A—Alcoholism, T*—Tumors, *I*—Idiopathic, *C*—Connective tissue disorders (e.g. amyloidosis)].

Clinical Stages or Features (Figs 1.18A and B)

Stage I: In this stage, pain is usually the presenting complaint and the patient complains of characteristic discomfort in the hand, but there is no precise localization to the median nerve. There may be history of morning stiffness in the hand.

Stage II: In this stage, symptoms of tingling and numbness, pain, paresthesia, etc. are localized to areas supplied by the median nerve.

Stage III: Here, the patient complains of clumsiness in the hand and impairment of digital functions, etc.

Stage IV: In this stage, sensory loss in the median nerve distribution area can be elicited and there is obvious wasting of the thenar eminence.

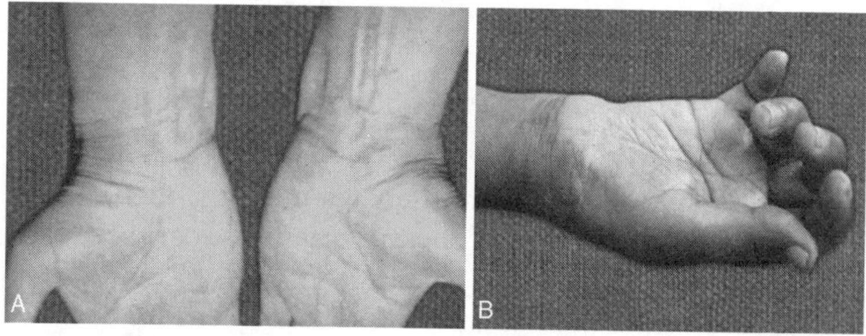

Figs 1.18A and B: (A) Clinical photograph of bilateral carpal tunnel syndrome, (B) Carpal tunnel (Clinical photo)

Clinical Tests

These are provocative tests and act as important screening methods and as an adjunct to the electrophysiological testing.

Wrist flexion (Phalen's test): The patient is asked to actively place the wrist in complete but unforced flexion. If tingling and numbness are produced in the median nerve distribution of the hand within 60 seconds, the test is positive. It is the most sensitive provocative test (Fig. 1.19). It has a specificity of 80 percent.

Tourniquet test: A pneumatic blood pressure cuff is applied proximal to the elbow and inflated higher than the patient's systolic blood pressure. The test is positive if there is paresthesia or numbness in the region of median nerve distribution of the hand. It is less reliable and is specific in 65 percent of cases only.

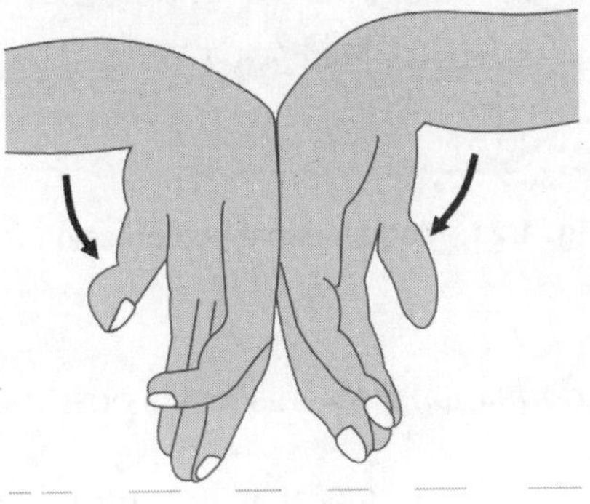

Fig. 1.19: Phalen's test

Median nerve percussion test: The examiner gently taps the median nerve at the wrist (Fig. 1.20). The test is positive if there is tingling sensation. Seen only in 45 percent of cases.

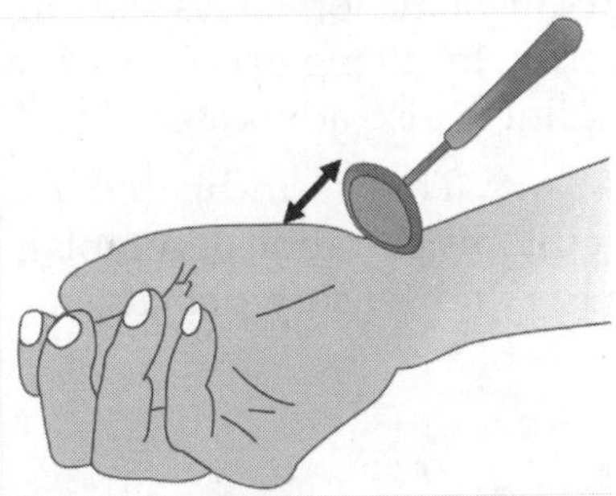

Fig. 1.20: Median nerve percussion test

Median nerve compression test: Direct pressure is exerted equally over both wrists by the examiner (Fig. 1.21). The first phase of the test is the time taken for symptoms to appear (15 sec to 2 min). The second phase is the time taken for the symptoms to disappear after release of pressure.

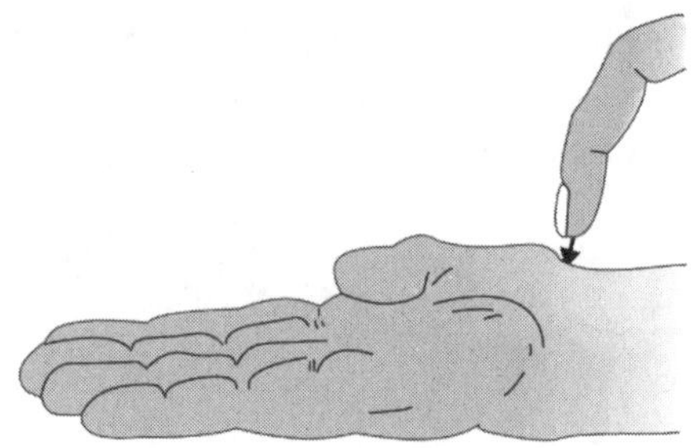

Fig. 1.21: Median nerve compression test

Other Tests

Two-point discrimination test: This test is positive in about one-third cases.

Electrodiagnostic tests are not very infallible with 10 percent individuals having normal values.

Treatment

Nonoperative methods: In the initial stages, non-steroidal anti-inflammatory drugs NSAIDs are given. If it is unsuccessful, steroids like prednisolone for 8 days starting with 40 mg for 2 days and tapering by 10 mg every 2 days are tried. Use of carpal tunnel splint is also advocated (Fig. 1.22).

Injection treatment: This is indicated in patients with intermittent symptoms, duration of complaints less than one year and if there is no sensory deficits, no marked thenar wasting, etc.

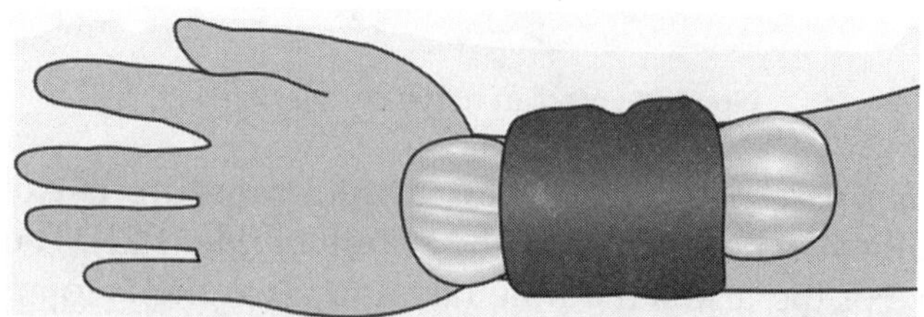

Fig. 1.22: Carpal tunnel splint

In the injection therapy, a single infusion of cortisone with splinting for 3 weeks is tried.

Surgery: This consists of division of flexor retinaculum and transverse carpal ligament and is indicated in failed nonoperative treatment, thenar atrophy, sensory loss, etc. (Fig. 1.23).

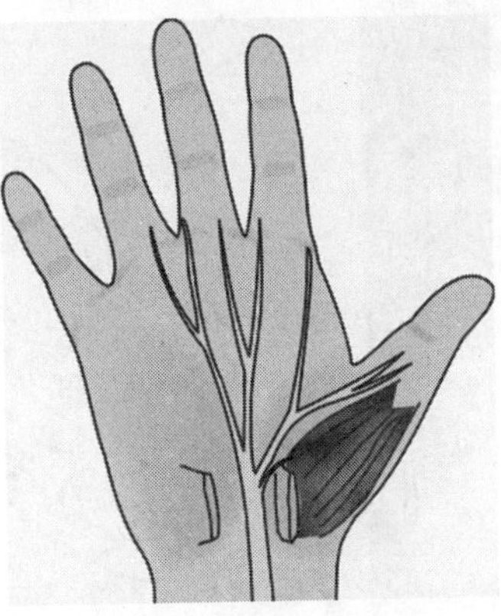

Fig. 1.23: Surgical division of the transverse carpal ligament

What is new in the treatment of carpal tunnel?

Chow's technique

This is an endoscopic release of the carpal ligament. It is a reliable alternative for the open procedure and has a success rate of 93.3 percent.

Percutaneous release of trigger fingers using a specially designed knife in difficult cases.

GANGLIA (GANGLION CYST)

The term *Ganglia* is derived from a Greek term meaning *Cystic tumor*.

Definition

It is defined as a localized, tense, painless, cystic, swelling, containing clear gelatinous fluid (Fig. 1.24A). It accounts for 50–70 percent of all soft tissue tumors of the hand and wrist.

Origin: The clear gelatinous fluid may be due to leakage or subsequent fibrous encapsulation of synovial fluid through the capsule of a joint or a tendon sheath (Fig. 1.24B).

Sites: It is commonly seen over dorsum of the wrist, flexor aspects of the fingers and dorsum of the foot.

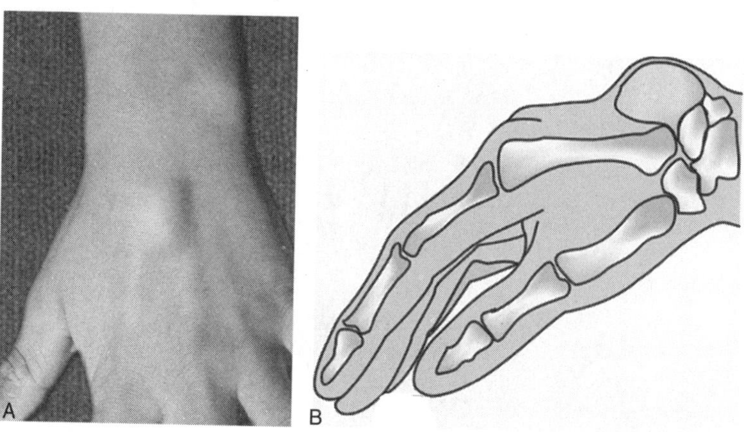

Figs 1.24A and B: (A) Clinical photograph showing a ganglion, (B) Origin of a ganglion

Quick facts: Ganglion

- Dorsal wrist ganglia accounts for 60–70 percent of all hand ganglia. It arises from scapholunate ligament.
- Volar ganglion—18–20 percent.
- Ganglion at the flexor tendon.
- Sheath at A1 pulley—10–12 percent.

Predisposing factors: Chronic repetitive stress and sometimes injury. It is more prevalent in women (M:F = 1:3).

Clinical Features

Swelling over the dorsum of the wrist is the only complaint. However, patient may complain of pain and enlarged swelling affecting the movements of the wrist in the event of complications.

Investigations

Plain X-ray of the part and laboratory examination of the aspirated fluid can be done.

Treatment

It may resolve spontaneously over a period. Excision is indicated if it is causing symptoms.

Biblical facts

What role the Holy Bible has in orthopedics? Well in ancient days, it was used to bang the ganglion into submission!

What is new?

Treatment of Ganglia: Arthroscopic release of the dorsal wrist ganglia is a sensible option than open excision for the following advantages:

- Minimal scarring
- Safe
- Faster rehabilitation
- Early mobility.

Did you know?

In some dorsal wrist ganglia is usually due to capsular abnormality in the region of interosseous scapholunate ligament.

NEUROVASCULAR CONDITIONS OF THE FOREARM

VOLKMANN'S ISCHEMIA OR COMPARTMENTAL SYNDROMES

Mubarak defined compartmental syndrome as an *elevation of interstitial pressure in a closed osseofascial compartment that results in microvascular compromise* and may cause irreversible damage to the contents of the space.

Sites

1. Anterior and deep posterior compartments of the legs.
2. Volar compartment of the forearm (Fig. 1.25).

3. Buttocks, shoulder, hand, foot, arm and lumbar paraspinous muscles are relatively rare sites.

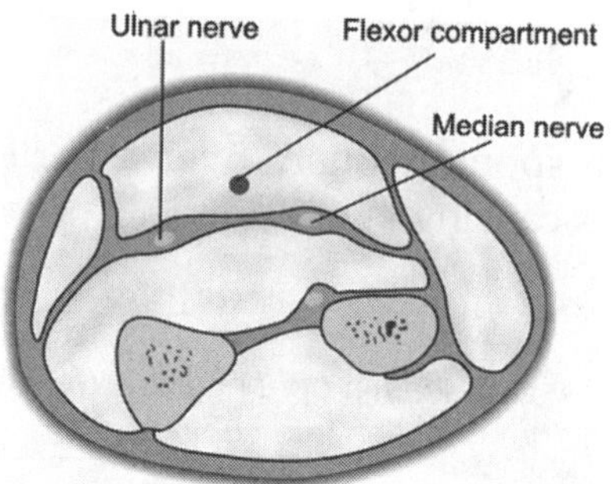

Fig. 1.25: Cross-section of the volar compartment of the forearm

COMPARTMENTAL SYNDROME OF FOREARM

This is one of the most dreaded complications in orthopedics and ranges from mild ischemia to severe gangrene. Early recognition and prompt remedial measures is the key to successful countering of this problem. *This is an orthopedic emergency.*

Definition

It is an ischemic necrosis of structures contained within the volar compartment of the forearm.

Incidence and Etiology

It is common in children less than 10 years of age.

- Supracondylar fracture is the most common cause in children.
- Crush injuries of the forearm are the most common causes in adults.
- Occasionally fracture of both bones of forearm dislocation of the elbow, vascular injuries and subfascial hematomas may be the cause.

- More recently intra-arterial injections in drug addicts who lie on their forearm for prolonged periods in narcotized conditions are mooted to be a cause (Fig. 1.26).
- Improper application of splints is another important cause.

Usually the flexor muscles of the forearm, especially the flexor digitorum profundus and flexor pollicis longus and rarely flexor digitorum superficialis are involved. Volkmann's ischemic contracture (VIC) is due to the infarction produced by an arterial spasm of the main artery to an extremity with reflex spasm of the collateral circulation. This produces ischemia of the muscle bellies that results in necrosis and is later replaced by fibrous tissue causing contractures.

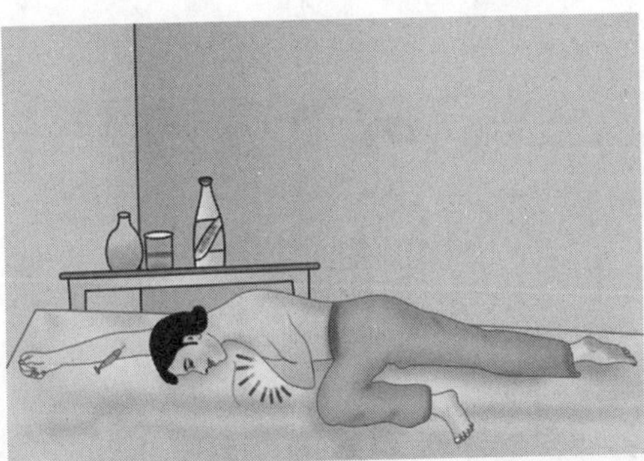

Fig. 1.26: Drug addicts 'beware' lying with your forearm tucked under your body in an inebriated state can lead to compartmental syndrome of the forearm

Pathology

An inelastic and unyielding deep fascia surrounds the forearm muscles. Rise in the intracompartmental pressure due to any cause is not accommodated and the vessels are compressed resulting in muscle ischemia and consequent fibrosis. The picture is one of *central* degeneration in the muscle along the line of anterior interosseous artery. The greatest damage is at the centre and the muscles commonly affected are flexor digitorum profundus and flexor pollicis longus.

Clinical Features

In the acute stages, the patient gives history of trauma and after an interval of few hours; severe, poorly localized pain develops in the forearm. The volar aspect of the forearm is swollen, red, warm, tender and tense. Fingers are held in flexion and an attempt to extend the fingers increases the pain (stretch pain) (Fig. 1.27). Peripheral pulses, which are present initially, disappear later. Median nerve is more commonly affected than the ulnar nerve.

> *Note:* In acute Volkmann's ischemia the patient complains of pain out of proportion to the injury.

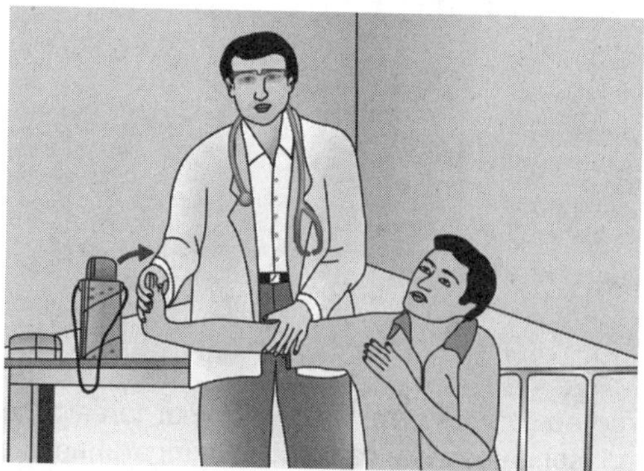

Fig. 1.27: Method of performing the passive stretch test

Impending Volkmann's ischemia is detected by 6Ps

- Pain
- Pallor
- Paresthesia
- Paralysis
- Pulselessness
- Positive passive stretch test.

Investigations

Investigations like routine blood tests, X-ray of the affected part, CT scan and MRI studies, angiograph and Doppler studies needs to be done before planning the treatment.

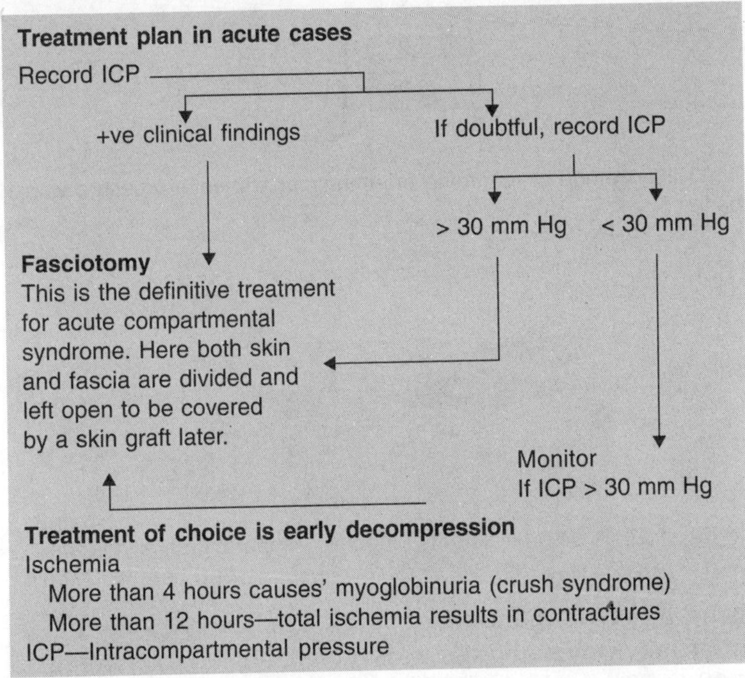

Management

Acute stage: It is a surgical emergency. All encircling tight bandages are removed, if present. If there is no improvement, record the pressure within the compartment (Fig. 1.28). If it is more than 30 mmHg, an emergency surgical decompression is done by fasciotomy (Fig. 1.29). If the pressure is less than 30 mmHg, continuous monitoring is done.

Methods to Record Intracompartmental Pressure

In any patient with forearm or leg injuries who has a tense compartment and if the patient is unreliable or unresponsive, the intracompartmental pressure should be recorded by

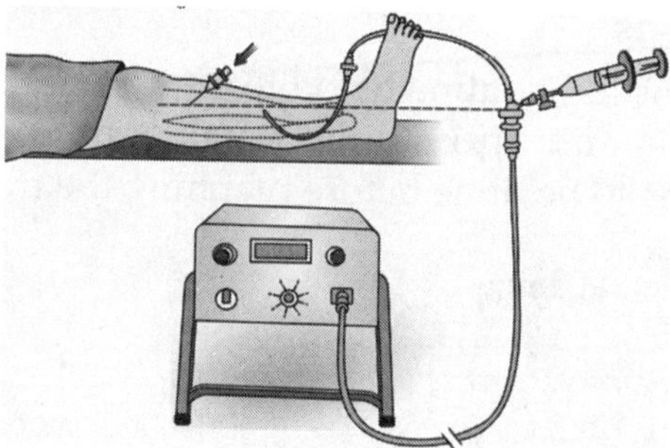

Fig. 1.28: Method of recording the intracompartmental pressure within the leg

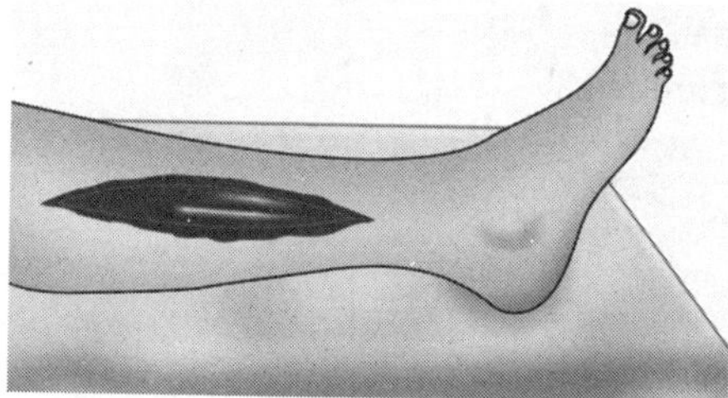

Fig. 1.29: A wide fasciotomy for acute compartmental syndrome

using a needle manometer, wick or slick catheter. If the intracompartmental pressure is more than 30 to 40 mmHg or is 10 to 30 mmHg more than the diastolic pressure of the patient, fasciotomy is recommended (Fig. 1.28).

Volkmann's Ischemic Contracture (VIC)

Late cases If mild, flexion contractures of flexor digitorum profundus and flexor pollicis longus develop but in severe cases all the finger flexors, thumb and wrist flexors are affected. The forearm is thin and fibrotic. Extensive scar tissue may be present. Peripheral nerves may be affected, amongst them median nerve is the most commonly involved. A *classical claw hand* deformity results (Fig. 1.30A) of particular importance is eliciting the *Volkmann's sign* in established VIC. *This test consists of extending the wrist, which* *exaggerates the deformities, and on flexion, the deformities appear less prominent (Figs 1.31A and B).* Joint contractures and gangrene may also be seen. Plain X-ray of the forearm shows old fracture (Fig. 1.30B).

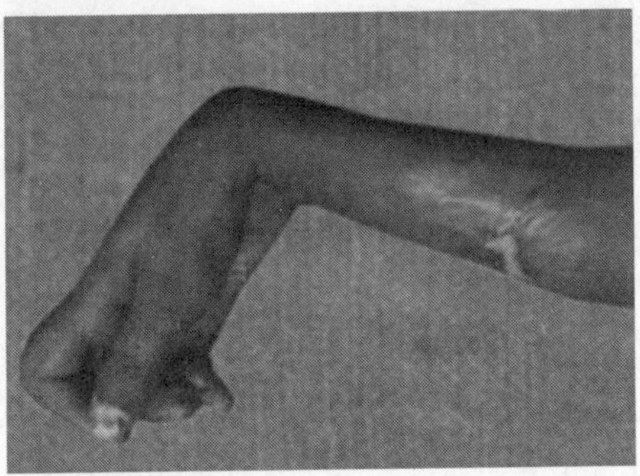

Fig. 1.30A: VIC of the forearm (Clinical photo)

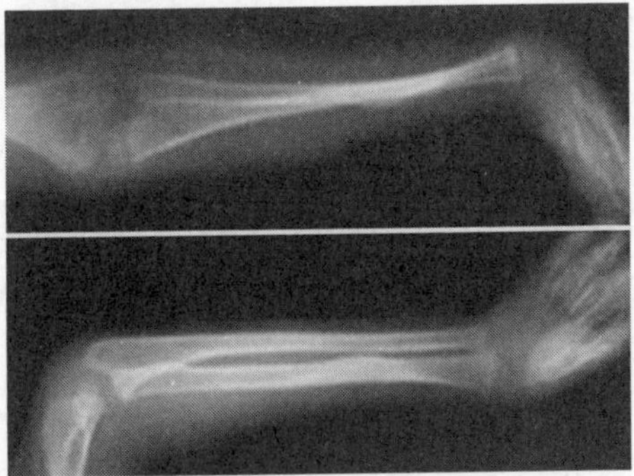

Fig. 1.30B: Radiograph of the VIC

In established VIC

Look for:

- Claw and deformity.
- Volkmann's sign.
- Extensive scarring of the forearm.
- Joint and soft tissue contractures.
- Neurological deficits.
- Rarely gangrene.

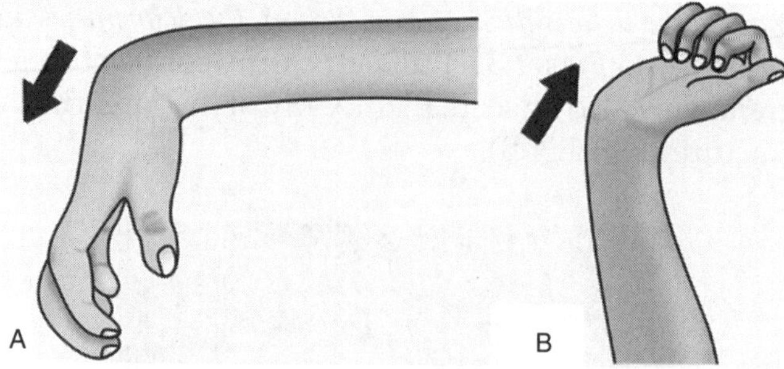

Figs 1.31A and B: Volkmann's sign: Deformity disappears on flexion (A) and appears on extension (B)

Remember

If 5 Ps help in detection of acute cases, 5 Ps also form clue to the management:

- Pressure to be relieved either external or internal.
- Pressure to be monitored within the compartment.
- Pulse to be recorded continuously.
- Passive stretch test indicates the severity.
- Putting the fracture back into its position.

Treatment Plan in Established VIC

Here the contractures are well-established and the treatment plan depends upon the severity of VIC.

Mild Type

- Dynamic splinting.
- Physiotherapy.
- Total excision if single muscle is involved.

Moderate Type

- *Max page's muscle sliding operation:* This consists of releasing the common flexor origin from the medial epicondyle and passively stretching the fingers. This slides the origin of the muscle down and releases the contractures.
- *Excision of cicatrix.*

- *Neurolysis:* It consists of freeing the peripheral nerves from the surrounding fibrous tissue.
- *Tendon transfers:* These are done if criteria are met.

Severe Type

- *Excision* of the scar.
- *Seddon's carpectomy*—It consists of excising the proximal row of carpal bones thereby shortening the forearm to overcome the effects of contracted muscles.
- *Arthrodesis* of the wrist in functional position.
- *Amputation* for very severe cases of VIC with gangrene.

Chronic Compartmental Syndrome

Chronic compartmental syndrome is a pretibial pain induced by exercise seen in the anterior compartment of the leg in athletes. If the compartmental pressure is more than 15 mmHg at rest, more than 30 mmHg during exercise and more than 20 mmHg for 5 minutes after exercise, chronic compartmental syndrome are suspected. Due to the herniation of fat or muscle through the fascial defect, a soft tissue mass is seen in the anterolateral aspect of the lower third of the leg. The patient is instructed to alter or decrease the level of activity, if no, if no relief is forthcoming, surgical decompression is indicated.

NEUROLOGICAL CONDITIONS OF THE FOREARM

ULNAR NERVE INJURY

Causes

General Causes

These are as described in the general principles of peripheral nerve injury.

Local Causes

These are more important and could be in the following areas:

Causes in the axilla

- Crutch pressure.
- Aneurysm of the axillary vessels.

Causes in the arm

- Fracture shaft of humerus.
- Gunshot and penetrating injuries.

Causes at the elbow

- Compression by the accessory muscle (anserina epitrochlearis).
- Fracture lateral epicondyle of humerus.
- Repeated occupational strains.
- Recurrent subluxation of the nerve.
- Compression by the osteophytes as in rheumatoid and osteoarthritis.
- Cubitus valgus deformity due to various causes results in repeated friction of the nerve giving rise to tardy (late) ulnar nerve palsy.

Causes in the forearm

- Fracture both bones forearm.
- Incised wounds, gunshot wounds and penetrating injuries of the forearm.

Causes at the wrist

- Compression by osteophytes.
- Fracture hook of the hamate.
- Compression by ganglion.
- Wrist injuries.

Causes in the hand

- Blunt trauma.
- Penetrating injuries.
- Occupational—people operating high-speed drills in rock mining, etc.
- Associated ulnar artery aneurysm.

Ulnar nerve injuries give rise to *clawhand* deformity either true type or ulnar clawhand.

CLAWHAND

It is a deformity with hyperextension of the metacarpophalangeal joints and flexion of the interphalangeal joints of the fingers.

Types and Causes

Two varieties are described: One is a true clawhand involving both median and ulnar nerves and the second an ulnar clawhand or claw-like hand due to ulnar nerve injury.

Pathomechanics

Loss of intrinsic muscle function due to ulnar nerve injury results in loss of flexion at MP joints and extension of IP joints of the fingers.

In a bid to bring about the flexion of the MP joints, the long finger flexors overact pulling the IP joints and wrist into more flexion. This causes a tenodesing (pulling) effect on the long finger extensors. The extensors cannot extend the IP joints without the stabilization of the MP joint in neutral or slightly flexed position, which is normally brought about by the intrinsic. This along with the compensatory over action of the long finger extensors to bring about the lost extension of the MP joints results in hyperextension of the MP joints and the classical deformity.

This is called the intrinsic minus hand: The thumb is also adducted by its long extensors because the intrinsics and the abductors are paralyzed.

Problems of clawhand

- Hyperextension of MP joints (not the only primary or most disabling deformity).
- Grasp decreased by 50 percent due to loss of power of flexion at MP joints.
- Pinch decreased due to loss of stabilizing effect from the intrinsics.
- Roll up maneuver lost.
  Many surgical procedures are devised to block hyperextension of MP joints as it is still considered as the primary deformity.

Note: MP—Metacarpophalangeal, IP—Interphalangeal.

Clinical Features

These include the classical deformity, loss of sensation along the ulnar nerve distribution and wasting of the hypothenar muscles, intrinsic muscles of the hand leading to hollow intermetacarpal spaces on the dorsum of the hand (Figs 1.32A to C).

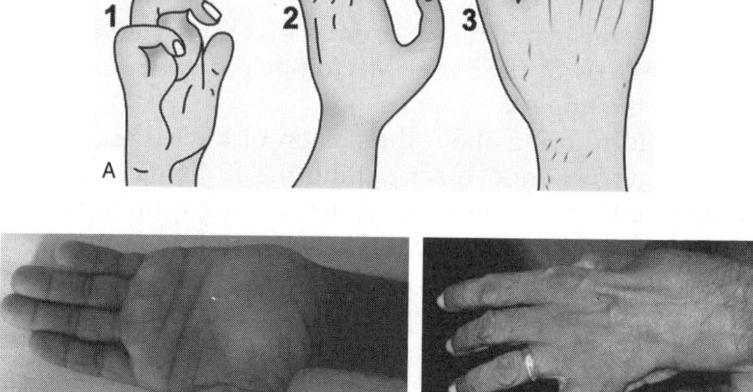

Figs 1.32A to C: (A) (1) Ulnar clawing, (2) Total clawing, and (3) Wasting of intermetacarpal spaces (B) Hypethenar muscle wasting (Clinical photo) (C) Intermetacarpal spaces (Clinical photo)

A test for loss of sensation along the distribution of the ulnar nerve in the hand and fingers is carried out. However, the clinical features vary depending upon the level of lesion.

Clinical Tests

For Ulnar Nerve Injury

Froment's sign: This is a reliable clinical test for ulnar nerve injury (Figs 1.33A and B). Three muscles (first palmar interossei, adductor pollicis and flexor pollicis longus) are required to hold a book between the thumb and other fingers. In ulnar nerve injury, the first two muscles are paralyzed and now to hold the book, the patient has to depend only on flexor pollicis longus, which flexes the thumb prominently. This is the positive Froment's sign.

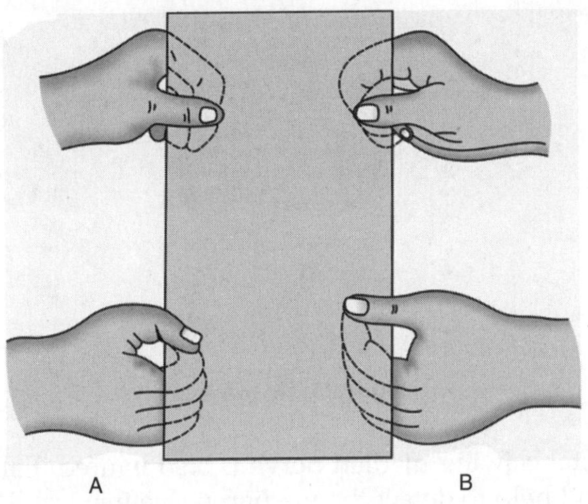

Figs 1.33A and B: Froment's sign: (A) Normal, (B) Ulnar nerve injury

Card test: Inability to hold a card or paper in between fingers due to loss of adduction by the palmar interossei (Fig. 1.34).

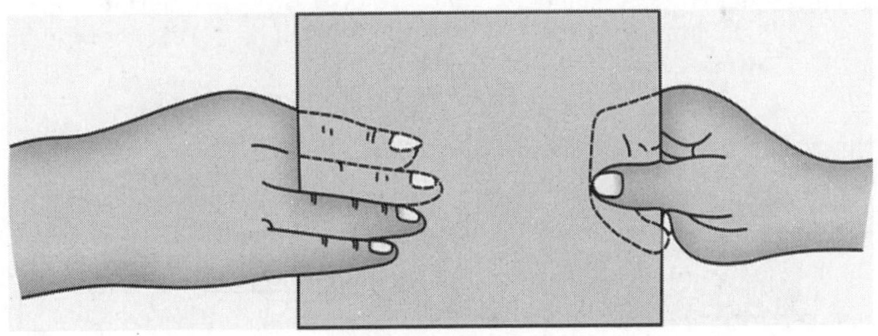

Fig. 1.34: Card test

Egawa test: With palm flat on the table the patient is asked to move the middle finger sideways (Fig. 1.35). This is a test for the dorsal interossei of middle finger.

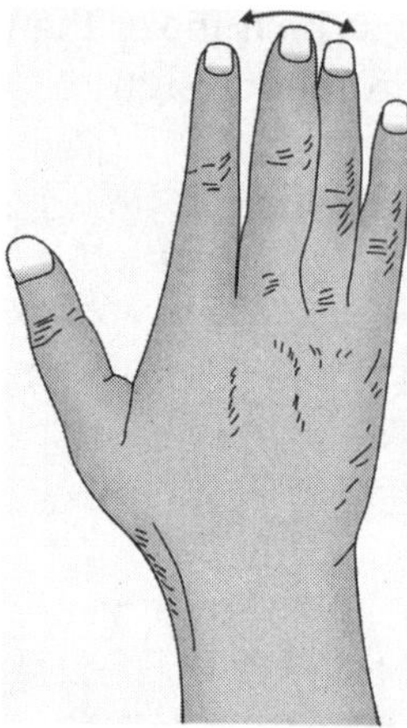

Fig. 1.35: Egawa test

In total clawing median nerve is also injured. Following tests will help to detect the median nerve injury.

Pen test: The patient is unable to touch the pen due to the loss of action of abductor pollicis brevis (Fig. 1.36).

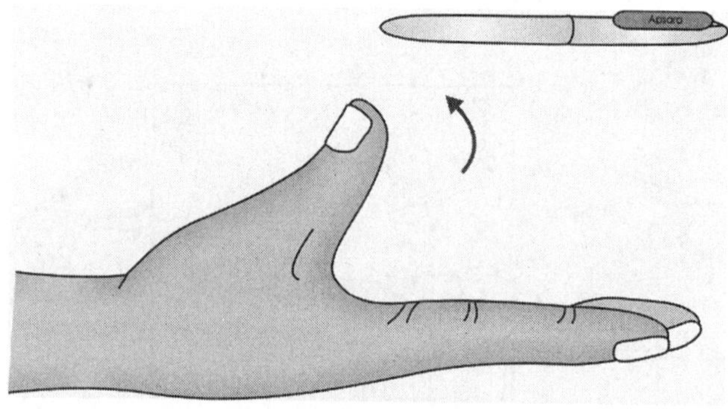

Fig. 1.36: Pen test

Pointing index or Oschner's clasp test: When both the hands are clasped together, index and middle fingers, fail to flex due to the loss of action of long finger flexors of the index and middle fingers, which are supplied by the median nerve (Fig. 1.37).

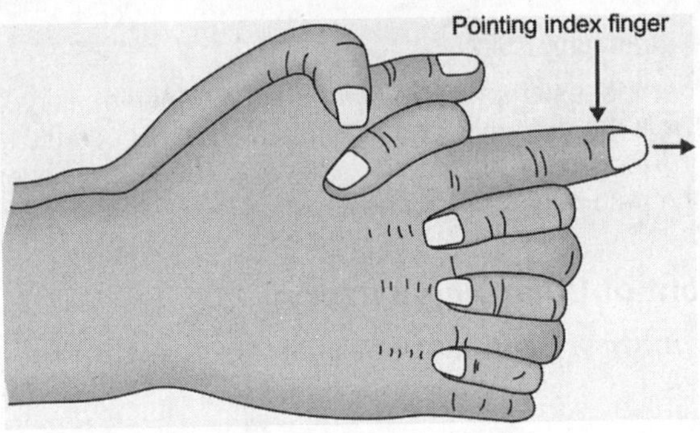

Fig. 1.37: Oschner's clasp test

Benediction test: For the same reason mentioned above, the patient is unable to flex the index and middle finger on lifting the hand (this is the position a clergyman uses to bless the couple during marriage (Fig. 1.38). Hence, called the benediction test).

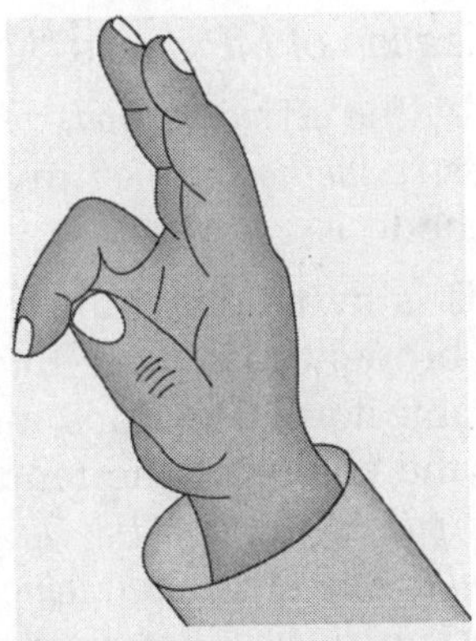

Fig. 1.38: Benediction test

Note: Median nerve supplies the following muscles:

- *In the forearm:* Pronator teres, flexor carpi radialis, palmaris longus, flexor digitorum superficialis, flexor digitorum profundus, flexor pollicis longus and pronator quadratus.
- *In the hand:* Abductor and flexor pollicis brevis, opponens pollicis middle and index lumbricals.

What is ulnar paradox?

The higher the lesion of the median and ulnar nerve injury, the less prominent is the deformity and vice versa. This is because in higher lesions the long finger flexors are paralyzed. The loss of finger flexion makes the deformity look less obvious.

Treatment of Ulnar Nerve Injury

In acute injuries, the treatment is as discussed in the general principles.

For Clawhand Deformity

Principles of treatment: All the treatment measures aim at blocking the hyperextension at the metacarpophalangeal joint. Once this joint is stabilized, the long extensors will bring about the extension of IP joints. The long finger flexors will help in flexion of the MP joints along with their action of finger and wrist flexion.

Methods of Stabilization of MP Joints

This can be done by the *active method, which involves tendon transfer,* or by *passive method, which* involves arthrodesis, capsulodesis or tenodesis.

Active method: This is by tendon transfers. A neighboring healthy tendon is brought to replace the action of the lost intrinsic. The available normal tendons and the existing local situations dictate the choice of the tendon. *Whichever the tendon chosen, it is passed through the lumbrical canal and is attached to the dorsal digital expansion, which then brings about the action of the lost intrinsics.* Before resorting to tendon transfers, certain criteria are to be followed.

Choice of Surgery

Modified S Bunnell's Operation

When finger flexors are strong, wrist flexors and extensors are strong, and if there is no habitual flexion of the wrist, modified S Bunnell's operation is preferred in which flexor digitorum superficialis of the ring finger is transferred through the lumbrical canal into the dorsal digital expansion.

Riordan's Operation

When flexion of the wrist has become habitual or if there is a flexion contracture of the wrist, a wrist flexor can be spared to overcome the above mentioned problems. In Riordan's operation, the flexor carpi radialis muscle is removed and transferred with a free tendon graft leaving behind the flexor carpi ulnaris to bring about the wrist flexion.

Brand's Operation

When the finger flexors are weak, the wrist flexors are also weak and when the wrist extensors are strong extensor carpi radialis longus or brevis is transferred by a free tendon graft.

Fowler's Operation

When finger flexors, wrist extensors and wrist flexors are not available for transfer, extensor digitorum longus tendon of the index and little fingers are transferred by the Fowler's technique.

When no muscle is available for transfer and if the joints are supple, capsulodesis of MP joint or tenodesis is done. If the joints are not supple, arthrodesis in functional position is done.

Tardy Ulnar Nerve Palsy

It is late onset ulnar nerve palsy and could be due to the following causes:

- Malunion or nonunion of lateral condyle fracture of humerus.

- Fracture medial epicondyle of humerus.
- Dislocation of elbow.
- Nerve contusions.
- Cubitus valgus.
- Shallow ulnar groove.
- Hypoplasia of humeral trochlea.
- Recurrent subluxation due to inadequate fibrous arch.

Treatment is by anterior transposition of the ulnar nerve.

ENTRAPMENT NEUROPATHY

Entrapment sites: The ulnar nerve could be entrapped in any one of the following sites during its anatomical course:

- Supracondylar process medially.
- Arcade of Stuther's (near medial intermuscular septum).
- Between two heads of flexor carpi ulnaris.
- Guyon's canal.

At a glance: Ulnar nerve injury

- Ulnar nerve root value is C_8T_1.
- Injury causes ulnar clawing.
- Total clawing when median nerve is also affected.
- Froment's sign is a reliable test.
- For quick clinical evaluation after injury, the tip of the little finger is tested for sensation.
- Ulnar paradox—higher the lesion less is the deformity and vice versa.
- Correction is by tendon transfers if all criteria are met.
- If no tendons are available for transfer, MP joint is stabilized by capsulodesis, tenodesis or arthrodesis.
- All surgeries aim at correcting the hyperextension at MP joint.

RADIAL NERVE INJURY

Causes

General

This could be due disease like leprosy, etc.

Local

In the axilla

- Aneurysm of the axillary vessels.
- Crutch palsy.

In the shoulder

- Proximal humeral fractures.
- Shoulder dislocation.

In the spiral groove 5′S

- Shaft fracture.
- Saturday night palsy (Fig. 1.39).
- Syringe palsy (Fig. 1.40).
- Surgical positions (Trendelenburg).
- 'S′march's (Esmarch) tourniquet palsy.

Saturday night palsy (Also called weekend palsy)

In this condition, there is compression of the radial nerve between the radiospiral groove and the lateral intermuscular septum.

It is known after an event which typically happens on a Saturday night weekend when in an inebriated condition, a person slumps with his mid-arm compressed between the arm of the chair and his body (Fig. 1.39).

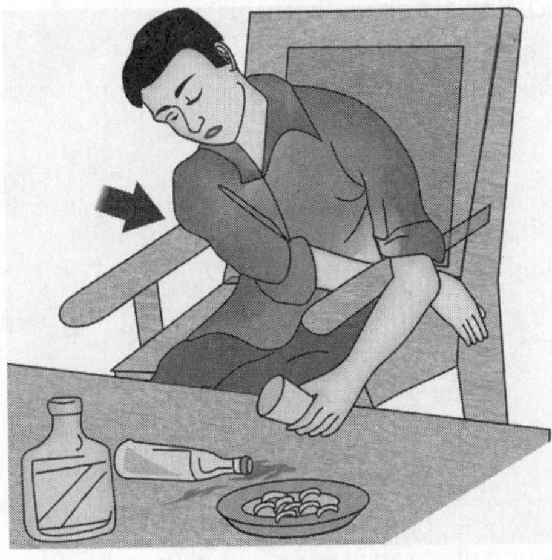

Fig. 1.39: Saturday night palsy (Patient's mistake)

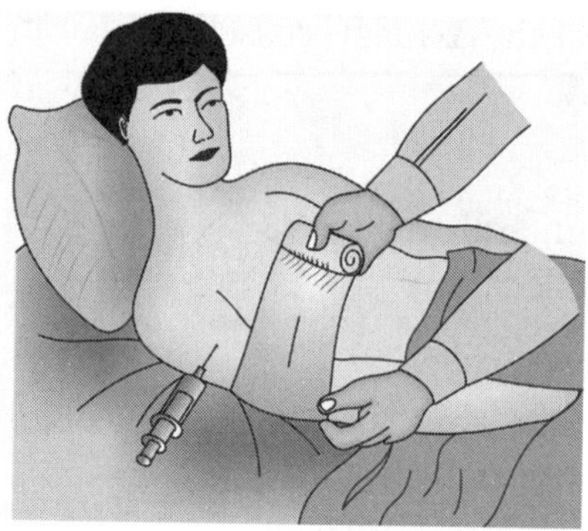

Fig. 1.40: Injection and tourniquet palsy (Doctor's mistake)

Did you know about honeymoon palsy?

- You have heard about Saturday night palsy, but have you heard about honeymoon palsy?
- Well, it is sleep palsy and is seen in young couples where a bed partner's head compresses the radial nerve, while resting in the crook of the partner's arms!

Between Spiral Groove and Lateral Epicondyle

- Fracture shaft humerus (Fig. 1.41).
- Supracondylar fracture humerus.

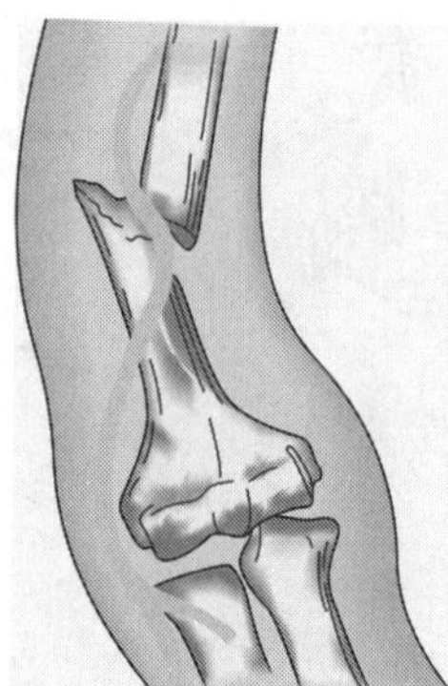

Fig. 1.41: Entrapment of radial nerve in between the fracture fragments of the humerus (nobody's mistake)

- Lateral epicondyle fracture of the humerus.
- Penetrating and gunshot injuries.
- Cubitus valgus deformity.

At the elbow

- Posterior dislocation of the elbow.
- Fracture head of radius.
- Monteggia's fractures.

Causes in the forearm

- Fracture both bones forearm.
- Penetrating and gunshot injuries.

Levels of lesion

	Features
High: Above spiral groove	Total palsy
Low: Type I *Between:* The spiral groove and the lateral epicondyle	*Spared:* Elbow extensor *Lost:* Motor • Wrist extensor • Thumb extensor • Finger extensors *Sensory:* Dorsum of first web space.
Low: Type II Below the elbow	*Spared* • Elbow extensor • Wrist extensor *Lost* : Motor • Thumb extensor • Finger extensor *Sensation* first web space

Clinical Features

If the lesion is high, the patient will present with wrist drop (Fig. 1.42), thumb drop and finger drop. He will be unable to extend the elbow. If the lesion is low the elbow extension is spared; but the wrist, thumb and the finger extensions are lost, but *the patient can extend the IP joints of the fingers because of the action of the intrinsic muscles of the hand*. Sensation along the posterior surface of the arm and forearm is lost in high

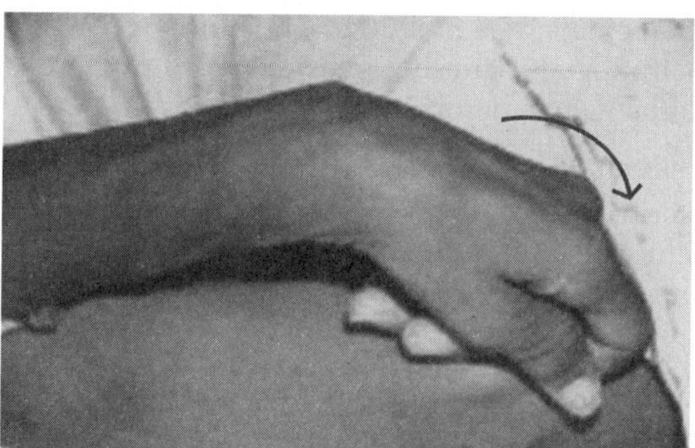

Fig. 1.42: Wrist drop (Clinical photo)

lesions and in low lesions the above sensations are spared, but there is loss of sensation over the first dorsal web space.

In acute injuries, it is difficult to evaluate the injury to the radial nerve. In such situations, the Hitchhiker's sign (inability to extend the thumb) is used as the screening test.

Investigations

Radiograph of the injured part and all other investigations mentioned in the general principles are carried out.

Treatment

Early cases: As mentioned in the general principles for closed fractures, conservative treatment is adopted. The patient is put on a cock-up splint or dynamic splints (Figs 1.43A and B). This is followed by active and passive physiotherapy. In failed conservative treatment, operative treatment is considered after a period of 12–18 months.

In open fractures, surgery is the treatment of choice. If the wound is clean, primary nerve repair is done, and if the wound is contaminated, delayed primary or secondary nerve repair is resorted to.

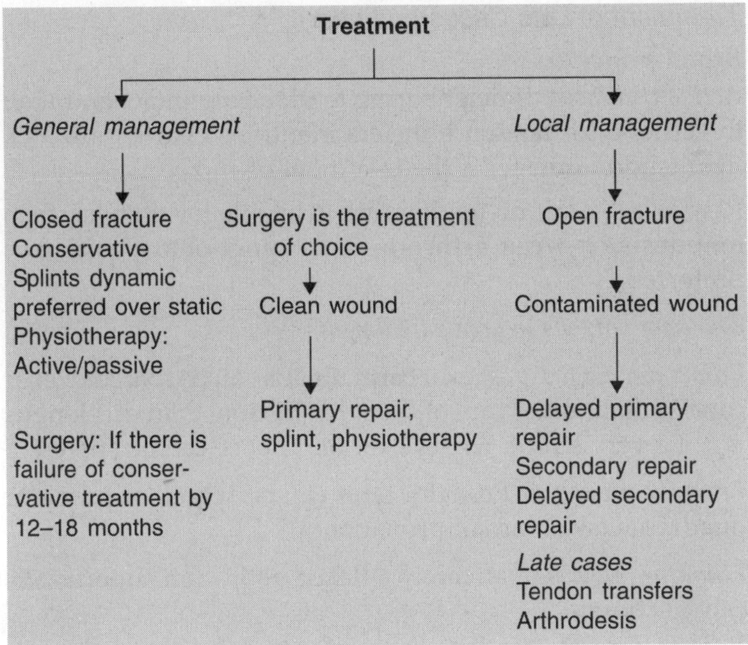

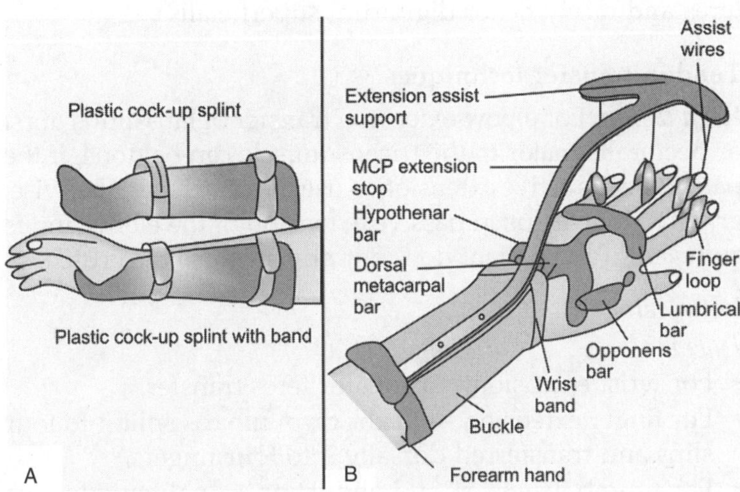

Figs 1.43A and B: Wrist drop splints: (A) Static or cock-up splint, (B) Dynamic splint

Treatment of Late Cases (> 1 year)

Broad principles

Active treatment: If neighboring tendons are intact and if all the criteria for tendon transfers mentioned earlier are met, then tendon transfer is the treatment of choice.

Passive method: If no tendons are available for transfer, then tenodesis or wrist arthrodesis in functional position is preferred.

Choice of tendons in active treatment

From the wrist flexors Flexor carpi ulnaris can be spared. Flexor carpi radialis takes care of the wrist flexion. Palmaris longus is not a very strong wrist flexor and hence can be spared.

From the pronators: Pronator teres can be spared as pronator quadratus takes care of pronation.

From the finger flexors, rarely a flexor digitorum superficialis can be chosen.

Therefore, the tendons chosen for transfer in radial nerve injuries are flexor carpi ulnaris, palmaris longus, pronator teres and rarely flexor digitorum superficialis.

Tendon transfer techniques

High lesion: For elbow extension transfer of latissimus dorsi or pectoralis major to the triceps muscle can be done, if the patient needs active extension to use the crutches. Otherwise, gravity alone helps in passive extension of the elbow and is sufficient if the patient does not prefer to use the crutches.

Low lesions

Type I

- For wrist extension → pronator teres transfer.
- For finger extension → flexor carpi ulnaris split into four slips and transferred dorsally into four fingers.
- For thumb extension and abduction → palmaris longus transfer.

Type II: Here wrist extension is spared and hence the plan is:

- For finger extension → flexor carpi ulnaris transfer (split into 4 slips).
- For thumb extension → palmaris longus transfer.
- For thumb abduction → pronator teres transfer.

Omer's technique: Consists of splitting flexor carpi ulnaris into five slips and transferring into all the five fingers instead of four.

Boye's technique: Uses flexor digitorum superficialis instead of flexor carpi ulnaris to bring about extension of four fingers.

Problems in radial nerve injury

- Wrist drop.
- Thumb drop.
- Finger drop only at MCP joint but extension at IP joint is possible due to action of interossei.
- Sensation over dorsal first web space is lost.
- In high lesions inability to extend the elbow and loss of sensations over posterior surface of arm and forearm are additional problems.

Radial nerve injury at a glance

- Continuation of posterior cord of the brachial plexus.
- Most common peripheral nerve to be injured.
- Most common site of injury is the distal end of humerus.
- Thumb extension test (Hitchhiker's sign) is the screening test.
- In radial nerve injury extension at finger IP joint is still possible.
- For early cases in closed fractures conservative treatment.
- For open fractures operative treatment and repair.
- For late cases, tendon transfers if neighboring tendons are available and if all the criteria are met.
- If no tendons are available, wrist arthrodesis is done in functional position.

Interesting nerve palsies concerning radial nerve

Did you know about handcuff palsy, dog handlers palsy or Cheiralgia paresthetica?

Well, all these are due to compression of the sensory branch of the superficial radial nerve at the level of the distal one-third of the forearm where it pierces the deep fascia and becomes dorsal.

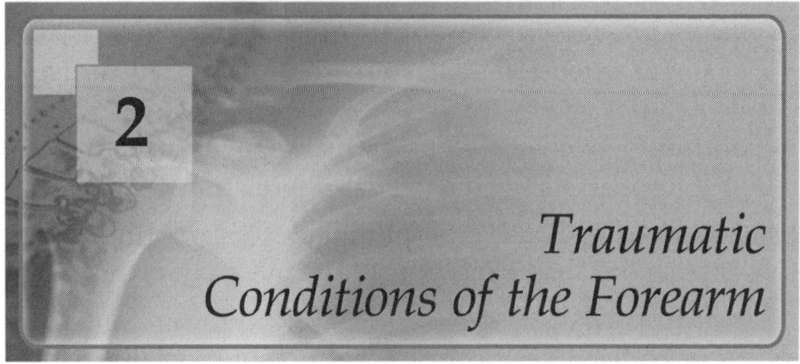

This chapter deals with important traumatic conditions of the forearm.

INJURIES OF THE FOREARM

Introduction

Injuries of the forearm present an interesting combination of injuries like fracture bones of forearm (Fig. 2.1), Monteggia's fractures, Galeazzi's fractures, Essex-Lopresti fracture, etc. The muscle attachments of the forearm make the treatment of these fractures difficult. The supinator muscle is inserted in the proximal third of the forearm bones and supinates this part of the forearm after the fracture. The middle third gives attachment to the pronator teres muscle and the distal third to the pronator quadratus. When the fracture occurs in the middle third, the forearm is held in the position of mid-pronation due to the balancing action of supinators and pronator quadratus muscle. In fractures of the distal third, the forearm is pronated due to the action of pronator quadratus. Hence, the treating physician should be aware of the various muscular forces (Fig. 2.2) acting in the forearm to effectively neutralize them and bring about proper union between the fracture fragments. Immobilizing the forearm in *supination* in upper third fractures, *midpronation* in middle third fractures and *pronation* in distal third fracture is found to effectively counter the muscular forces, which threaten to displace the fracture fragments.

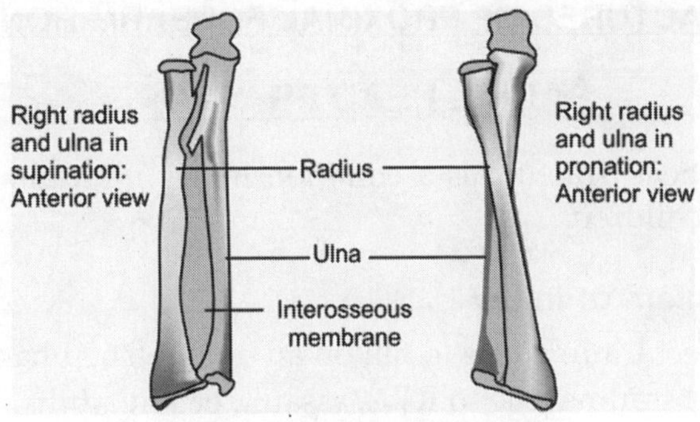

Fig. 2.1: Bones of the forearm

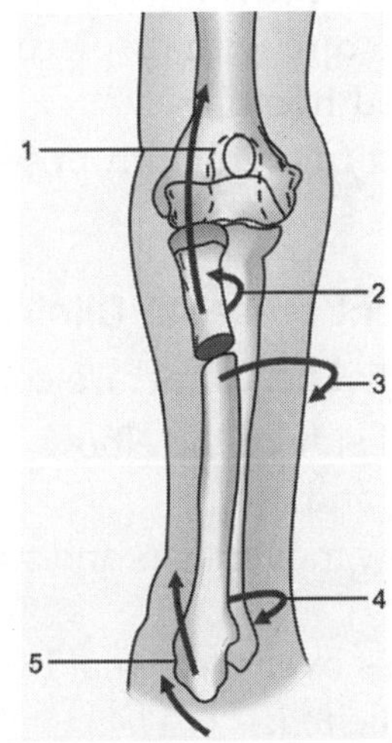

Fig. 2.2: Muscle forces in fracture both bones of forearm: (1) Biceps, (2) Supinator, (3) Pronator teres, (4) Pronator quadratus, and (5) Brachioradialis

Monteggia's fracture along with Galeazzi's fracture forms a rare and interesting combination of injuries where there is fracture of one bone with dislocation of the other. Curiously both are described in the forearm with the former involving the upper and middle forearm, and the latter involving the distal forearm.

FRACTURES OF PROXIMAL FOREARM BONES

RADIAL HEAD FRACTURE

Radial head fracture is a common injury in adults and is rare in children.

Mechanism of Injury

- Indirect trauma due to fall on an outstretched hand.
- Direct trauma due to RTA, assault, etc. in adults.

Mason's Classification (For medical readers only)

Type I: Undisplaced fracture.
Type II: Marginal fracture with displacement.
Type III: Comminuted fractures.
Type IV: Radial head fracture with posterior dislocation of elbow.

How does the patient present? Clinical Features

The patient with radial head fracture complains of:

- Pain on the lateral side of the elbow
- Minimal swelling and
- Restriction of elbow movements and supination pronation of the forearm.
- There is tenderness over the radial head and
- Crepitus can be elicited.

Investigation

Plain X-ray of the elbow including the antero-posterior and lateral radiographs of the elbow (Figs 2.3A and B).

Additional oblique radiograph delineates the fracture line better. CT scan helps to delineate the fracture pattern better.

Methods of Management: Treatment

This varies according to the type of fractures and ranges from simple immobilization of the elbow with sling or splint

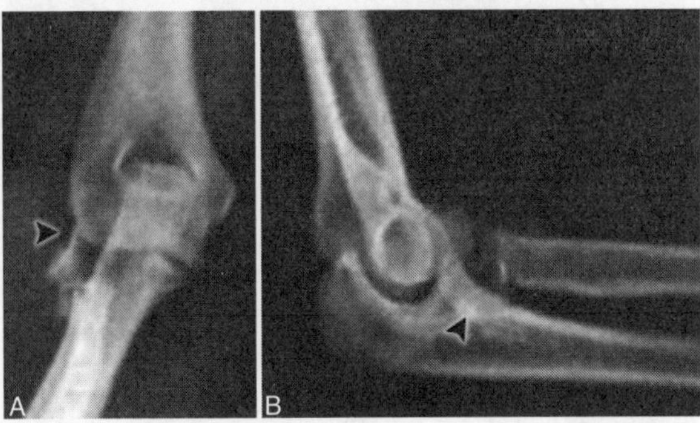

Figs 2.3A and B: Radial head fracture complete

and open reduction or excision of the comminuted radial head fragments.

Radial head replacement is controversial since excision of the head is usually effective in isolated comminuted radial head fracture that too if the medial collateral ligament is intact (Fig 2.4). However, metal radial head replacement is superior to silicone prosthesis.

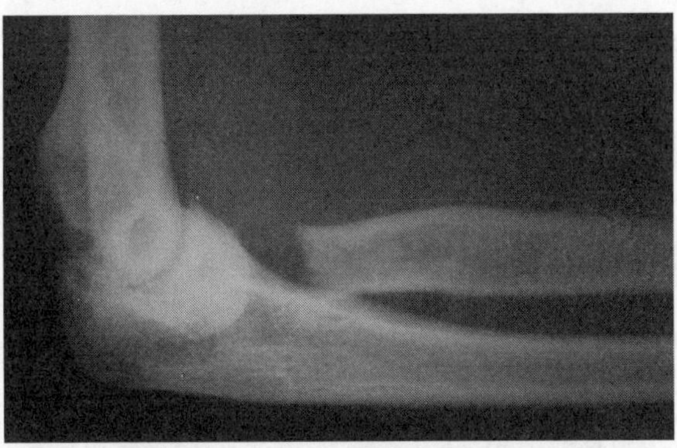

Fig. 2.4: Excision of the radial head

Complications

- Injury to the posterior interosseous nerve,
- Osteoarthritis and
- Elbow stiffness

Mystifying facts

Radial head excision does not cause instability (due to the presence of interosseous membrane) or functional impairment (due to the distal radioulnar joint).

FRACTURE OF THE OLECRANON

Introduction

Fracture olecranon is uncommon in children. Olecranon fracture in adults is comparable to fracture patella. Fracture reduction should be exact since any residual irregularity of the articular surface will cause limited motion, delayed recovery and traumatic arthritis of the elbow.

The fracture fixation should be strong enough to allow gentle active exercises even before radiographs show evidence of complete union.

As separation of the fracture of the patella causes quadriceps insufficiency so does displaced fracture olecranon causes triceps insufficiency.

Mechanism of Injury

Direct: Trauma due to fall on the point of elbow. This is the frequent cause (Fig. 2.5).

Indirect: Due to forcible triceps contraction.

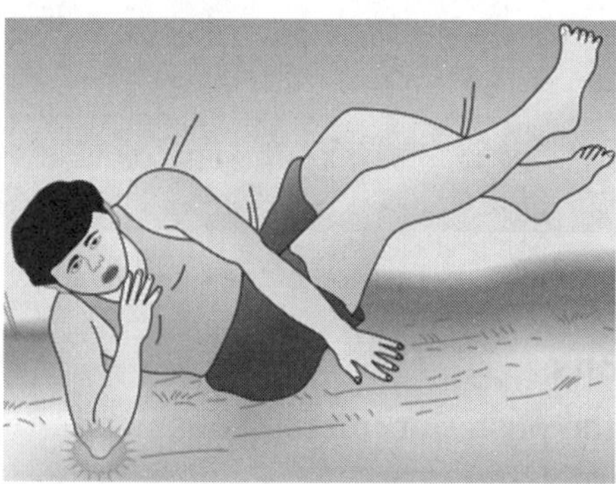

Fig. 2.5: Most common mechanism of olecranon fracture

Colton's Classification (Figs 2.6A to C) (Modified Schtazker) (For medical readers only)

- Undisplaced fracture
- Displaced fracture
- Avulsion fracture
- Transverse/oblique fracture
- Fracture dislocation (Monteggia group)
- Comminuted fracture.

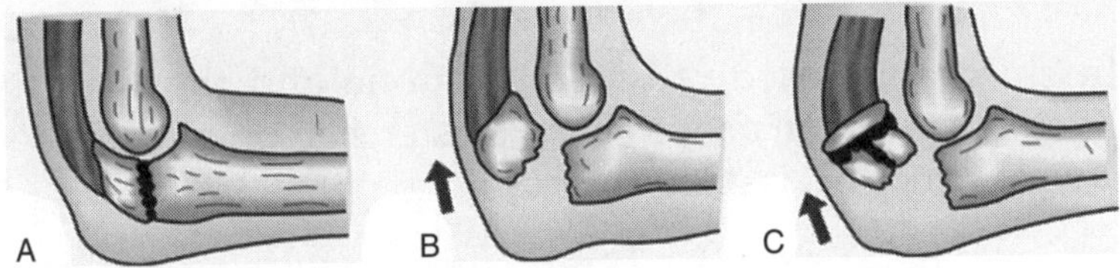

Figs 2.6A to C: Undisplaced fractures: (A) Displaced, (B) Comminuted, and (C) Fracture of olecranon

How does the patient present? Clinical Features

The patient complains of:

- Pain around the elbow
- Swelling ranging from mild to gross
- Inability to extend the elbow
- Tenderness and
- Crepitus can be elicited.

Radiographs

Routine anteroposterior and lateral views of the elbow help in confirmation of the diagnosis (Figs 2.7A and B).

> *Note:* In olecranon fracture more than 2 mm separation between fracture fragments is called displaced fracture.

Treatment

Conservative

Indications: This is indicated for undisplaced fractures and in fractures with less than 2 mm displacement.

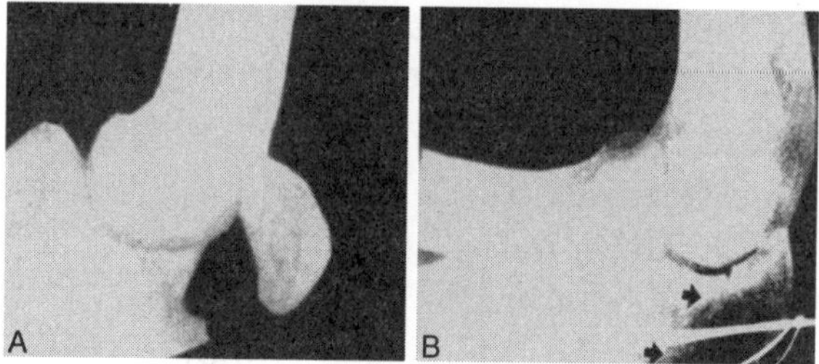

Figs 2.7A and B: Radiographs showing olecranon fracture and fixation with TBW

In children, closed reduction is done and the limb is immobilized in an above elbow plaster slab or cast for 3 to 4 weeks and this is often successful.

Surgery

In adults, repair of triceps is done for avulsion fractures. There is no place for conservative treatment, because closed reduction needs immobilization in extension for 6 to 8 weeks, which except in children causes permanent stiffness. Hence, surgery is the treatment of choice in adults.

Methods of operative treatment

Open reduction and internal fixation with figure of '8' wire loop (Figs 2.8A and B): This method is used for avulsion and

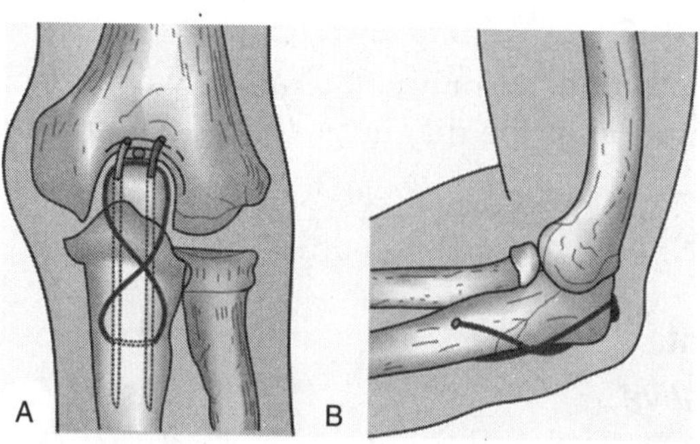

Figs 2.8A and B: Tension band wiring (TWB) in fracture olecranon

transverse fractures of the olecranon and for fractures which are uncomminuted and proximal to the coronoid fossa.

Medullary fixation by a single interfragmentary screw: This is indicated in comminuted fracture of olecranon when its distal fragment and the head of the radius are dislocated anteriorly. Rigid fixation is required to prevent recurrence of dislocation.

Excision of the proximal fragments

Indications

- In comminuted fractures.
- In delayed union or nonunion of fractures in upper half.
- If the patient is greater than 50 years of age and is not involved in heavy work.

This method is useful only if enough of the olecranon is left to form a stable base for the trochlea. Thus, it is not indicated when comminution extends as far as the coronoid.

Combination of intramedullary pin or screw and tension bands.

Contoured plate and screws are indicated in comminuted fractures with bone loss where tension band wiring cannot be done.

Disturbing facts

Reoperation rate after tension band wiring in olecranon fracture is as high as 71.7 percent due to backing out of the K-wire.

Complications

- Nonunion of the fracture,
- Osteoarthritis of the elbow,
- Triceps insufficiency and
- Restricted movements of the elbow are the common complications of fracture olecranon.

When do you consider olecranon fracture as stable?

If after reduction it does not separate or if the separation does not increase with flexion of elbow to 90°.

Quick facts

Treatment of displaced olecranon fractures concisely:

- Avulsion fracture—TBW/LS
- Transverse fractures—TBW/LS
- Transverse fractures with—Plate and screws with bone grafting
- Oblique fractures—LS/Plate
- Comminution—Excision/plate/TBW
- Fracture dislocation—Wire/LS/Plate

TBW—Tension band wiring
LS—Lag screw fixation.

CORONOID FRACTURES

Introduction

Fractures of the coronoid process of the ulna were earlier thought to be an avulsion fracture involving the brachialis muscle. Of late, this notion has been dispelled as it is found that the insertion of this muscle is more distal.

Interesting facts about coronoid fractures

- Its presence indicates a significant trauma to the elbow.
- It also points towards the possibility of acute recurrent dislocations.

Mechanism of Injury

This fracture occurs due to the impact of the coronoid process against the trochlea following a fall on an outstretched hand.

Classification of Regan and Morrey (Fig. 2.9A)
(For medical readers only)

Type I: Avulsion fracture of the tip of the coronoid.

Type II: Fracture involving greater than 50 percent of the coronoid.

Type III: Fracture involving the base of the coronoid.

Clinical Features

Isolated fractures of the coronoid process are usually rare and are usually associated with greater elbow trauma.

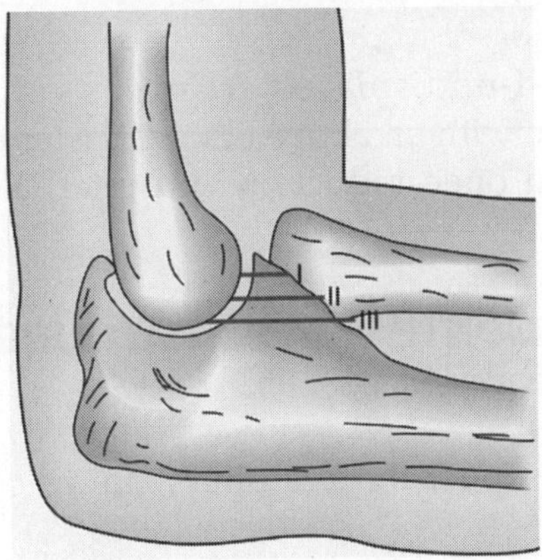

Fig. 2.9A: Types of coronoid fractures

Clinical features like

- Pain,
- Swelling,
- Deformity,
- Movement restriction of the elbow, etc. Depends on the extent of damage.

Radiograph

This fracture can be easily identified over a true lateral X-ray of the elbow (Fig. 2.9B).

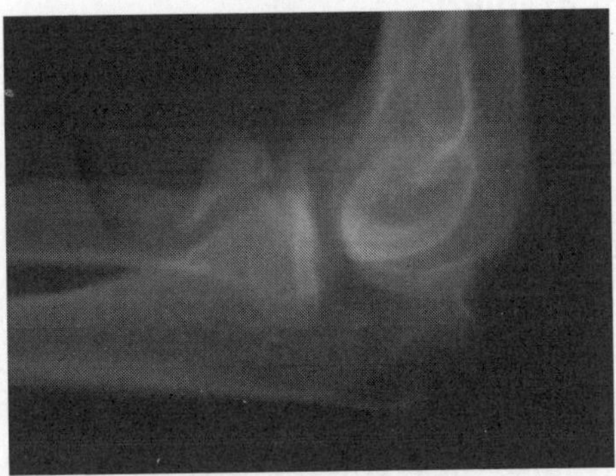

Fig. 2.9B: Radiograph of coronoid fracture

Treatment

Though small-undisplaced fractures can be managed conservatively with an above elbow plaster cast, displaced fractures need open reduction and internal fixation with screw or wires.

MONTEGGIA'S FRACTURE

Introduction

It is a fracture upper third of ulna with dislocation head of the radius.

This is usually called a "treacherous lesion" because the dislocation is often missed (see box for the reasons).

Monteggia first described it in 1881.

Monteggia's fractures, why called as treacherous.

Because dislocation of the head of the radius is often missed.

Reasons

- *Missed by patient*: As he reflexly pulls the elbow after fall and reduces the dislocation unknowingly.
- *Missed by quack* due to ignorance.
- *Missed by physician:* Fails to order to include the elbow in radiographs of forearm bone fractures.
- *Missed by radiologist:* If he or she fails to utilize the McLaughlin's line.

Mechanism of Injury

Monteggia's fractures are more common in children and are due to fall on the outstretched hands either in hyperpronation or in hyperextension (Fig. 2.10).

Classification (For Medical readers only)

Bado's classification is employed in adults and John Wein's classification in children and which takes into consideration the greenstick fractures in them (Figs 2.11A to E).

Monteggia's equivalents: These are variants of Monteggia's fracture dislocations and are a result of pronation injuries.

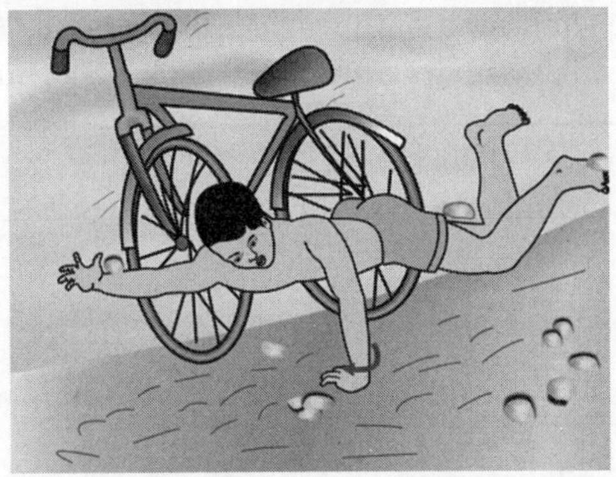

Fig. 2.10: Hyperpronation injury leading to fractures like Monteggia's

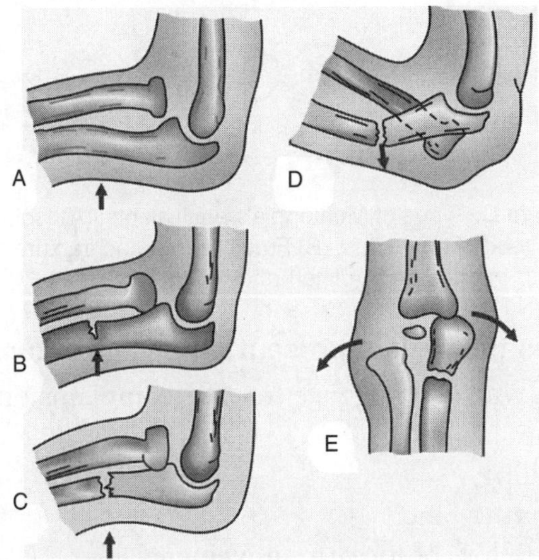

Figs 2.11A to E: Diagrammatic representation of the displacements in Monteggia's fracture; **Bado's Types** (Adults) C-type I, D-type II, E-Type III; **John Wein's Types** (Children). (A) Anterior bend, (B) Anterior greenstick, and (C) Anterior complete

The following types are described:

- Isolated dislocation of head of the radius.
- Fracture shaft ulna with fracture neck radius.

- Fracture shaft ulna with fracture shaft radius (distal).
- Fracture ulna with fracture radial neck, dislocation of shaft of the radius.

In these cases, closed reduction is tried first. If it fails, open reduction and internal fixation is done (Figs 2.12A to C).

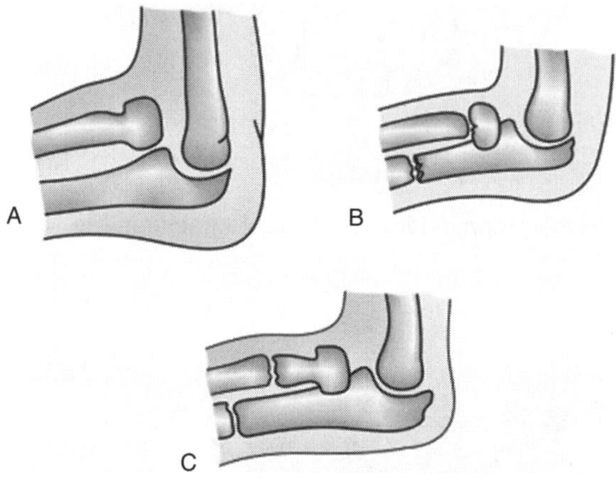

Figs 2.12A to C: Types of Monteggia's equivalents: (A) Isolated anterior dislocation head of the radius, (B) Fracture ulna and fracture neck radius, and (C) Both fracture ulna (distal) and radius (proximal)

How does the patient present? Clinical Features

A patient with Monteggia's fracture complains of

- Pain,
- Swelling,
- Deformity and
- Severe loss of forearm movements.
- Depending upon the type of Monteggia's fractures the head of the radius and the ulnar angulation may be felt anteriorly, posteriorly or laterally.

Radiographs

Plain X-ray of the forearm AP, lateral and oblique views including both the elbow and wrist joints needs to be done (Figs 2.13A to C).

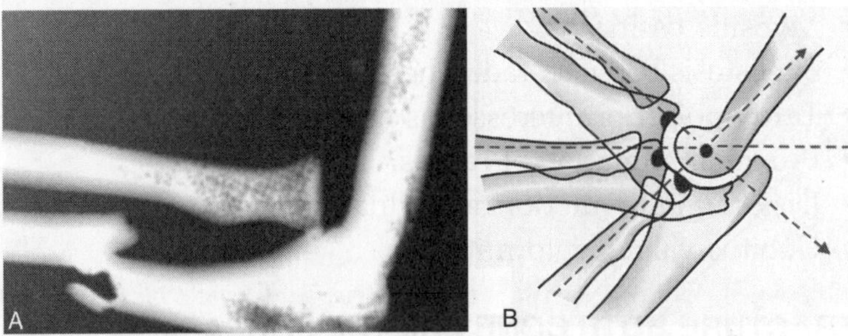

Figs 2.13A and B: (A) Radiograph showing Monteggia's anterior fracture, and (B) McLaughlin's line

In order to avoid missing the diagnosis of dislocation of the head of radius, McLaughlin's line is employed as described below (Figs 2.13B).

A straight line drawn along the center of the shaft of the radius cuts the capitulum in the center irrespective of the position of the elbow.

Treatment

Monteggia's fracture can be managed successfully in children by conservative methods like closed reduction and immobilization with plaster casts and by operative methods in adults consisting of open reduction and internal fixation with plate and screws.

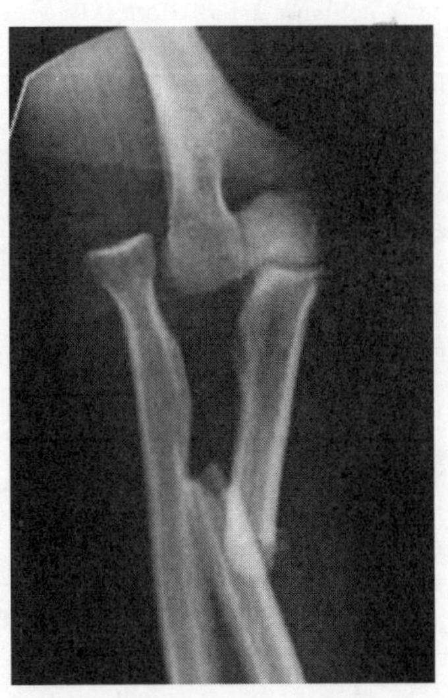

Fig. 2.13C: Radiograph of lateral Monteggia

Complications

- Unreduced dislocation head of radius.
- Posterior interosseous nerve palsy.
- Malunion of fracture ulna.
- Nonunion of fracture ulna.

- Myositis ossificans.
- Synostosis between radial head and proximal ulna.
- Tardy posterior interosseous nerve palsy.
- Proximal migration of radius.
- Dislocation of inferior radioulnar joint.
- Cubitus valgus deformity.

FRACTURE BOTH BONES OF THE FOREARM

Mechanism of Injury

Fracture both bones of forearm in adults are frequently due to RTA, falls, assault, etc. This is a difficult problem especially in adults. The complex muscle arrangements already described makes retention of the fracture fragments very difficult. The fracture could be due to either direct or indirect trauma (Figs 2.14A to C).

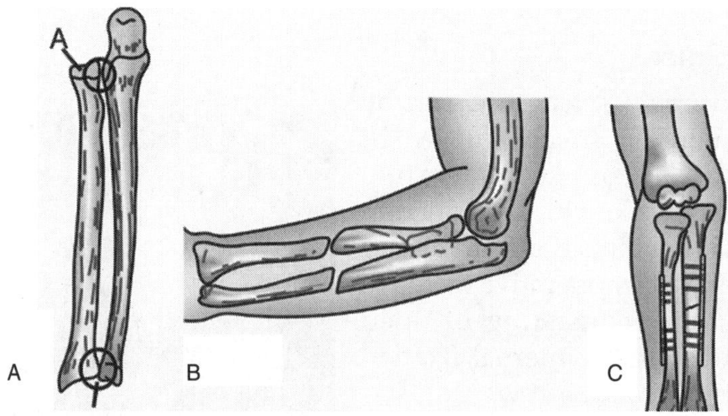

Figs 2.14A to C: (A) Normal both bones of the forearm with superior and inferior radioulnar joints, (B) Fracture both bones of the forearm, and (C) Fracture both bones fixed rigidly with plate and screws (Preferred method)

How does the patient present: Clinical Features

The patient presents with

- Severe pain,
- Swelling and

- Deformity of the forearm.
- Movements of the forearm are severely restricted and all other features of fractures are usually present.

Radiographs

The AP, lateral and oblique views of the forearm help to make an accurate diagnosis (Fig. 2.15A).

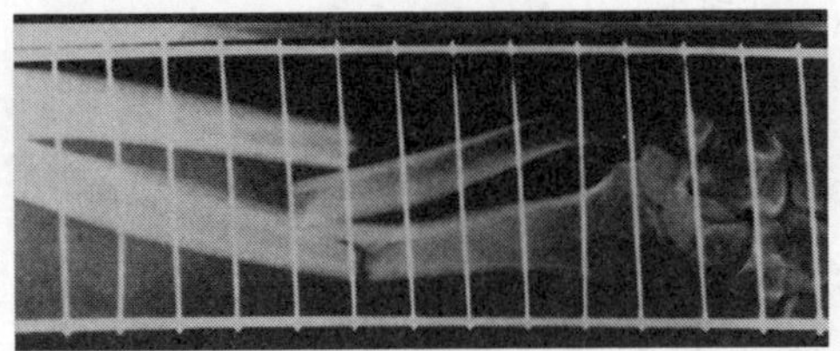

Fig. 2.15A: Radiograph showing fracture of radius and ulna

How to manage these injuries? Treatment

Conservative treatment: Undisplaced, incomplete fractures are treated by immoblilization with an above elbow plaster slab or cast. The treatment for displaced fractures consists of closed reduction by traction and counter traction methods under general anesthesia followed by an above elbow plaster cast, is usually successful in children.

Surgery: In adults ORIF is often indicated because it is difficult to regain length, apposition, axial and normal rotational alignment in adults by closed reduction. Open reduction is by two approaches, one for the radius and the other for the ulna (Fig. 2.15A). The choice of implants for ulna is either a medullary nail or plate and screws but for fracture radius, rigid compression plating is usually desired (Figs 2.14C and 2.15B). Cancellous bone grafting is done if the comminution is more than one-third of the circumference of the bone.

The choice of plate osteosynthesis are:

- Dynamic compression plates are still popular.

- *Low contact:* DCP have the advantage of less periosteal vascular damage.
- DCP plates with preliminary K-wire fixation helps in holding the fracture reduction while the final screws are fixed.
- *Low contact:* Locking dynamic compression plates helps to obtain both rigid fixation and less vascular damage.
- Locked compression plating is the preferred method of late.

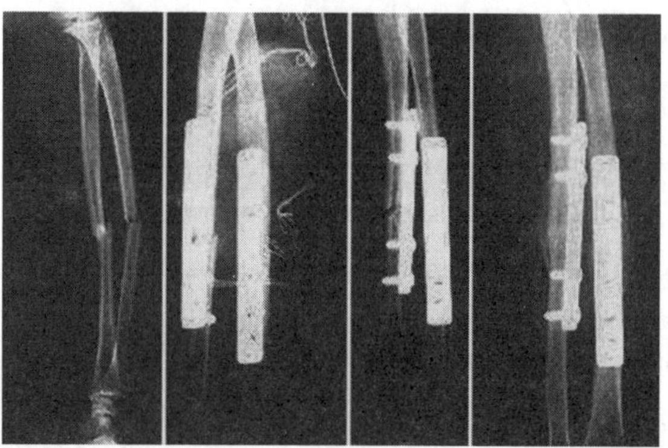

Fig. 2.15B: Radiograph showing forearm both bones fracture and internal fixation with DCP plates

Intramedullary fixation: IM nail fixation of both bones fractures with K-wires, Rush nails, etc. was popular in the 1950s and was gradually replaced by plates due to the less rigid fixation it offered. Now they are coming back with a bang. Thanks to the innovations in the nails technology like the advent of intramedullary interlocking nailing and is being mainly used in the pediatric group than adults.

Indications

- Segmental fracture
- Open fracture with soft tissues injury and/or bone loss
- Multiple injuries
- Failed plating
- Pathological fractures.

Advantages

- Less exposure
- Less periosteal stripping
- Bone grafting is not required

Choices of IM Nails

- Nonreamed interference fit, prebent star shaped titanium radial and ulnar nails.
- Stainless steel straight distal locking nail system.
- Interlocking nails with both proximal and distal locking.

What are the problems of these fractures?
Complications of Fracture Both Bones of Forearm

Volkmann's ischemia: Because of the tight fascial compartment, a patient with fracture both bones forearm is more prone to develop acute compartmental syndrome.

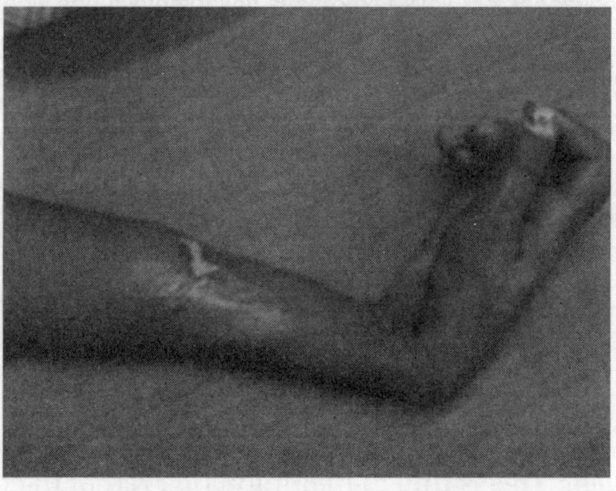

Fig. 2.16A: Clinical picture of VIC

Delayed union and nonunion: This can be encountered due to soft tissue interposition, inadequate immobilization, etc. It has to be treated by open reduction, rigid internal fixation and cancellous bone grafting.

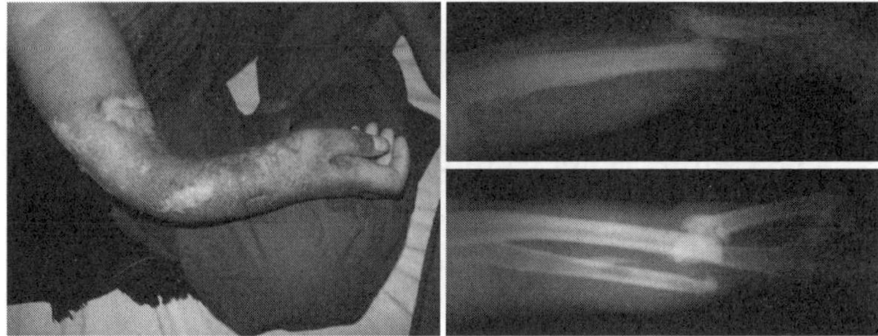

Fig. 2.16B

Malunion: Due to the complex muscular forces it is difficult to retain the position of both bones in perfect alignment after closed reduction. It is in this situation that malunion commonly results. It is treated by corrective osteotomy, plating and bone grafting.

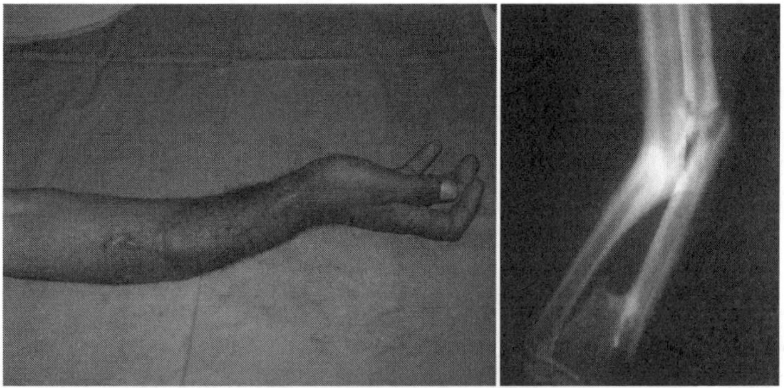

Fig. 2.16C

Cross union: This is due to malunion of a radial fracture in a medially deviated position, which occupies the interosseous space and blocks pronation and supination. If the crossunion takes place in the middle third of the forearm, it can be left alone as the forearm is held in midpronation with less functional damage. Elsewhere, it needs corrective osteotomy and rigid internal fixation.

ISOLATED DISTAL ULNAR FRACTURE

This is also called nightstick fracture and is relatively rare when compared to fracture both bones of the forearm.

It is usually due to direct blow on the subcutaneous border of the ulna (Fig. 2.17A). Three types are described:

Type I: Simple fracture.

Type II: Comminuted fracture without distal radioulnar joint involvement.

Type III: Type II with involvement of the distal radioulnar joint.

Interesting facts

Nightstick fracture derives its name from the peculiar incident of a burglar getting caught during his misadventure in the night and trying to ward off the police officer's blow with the stick with his forearm (Fig. 2.17A).

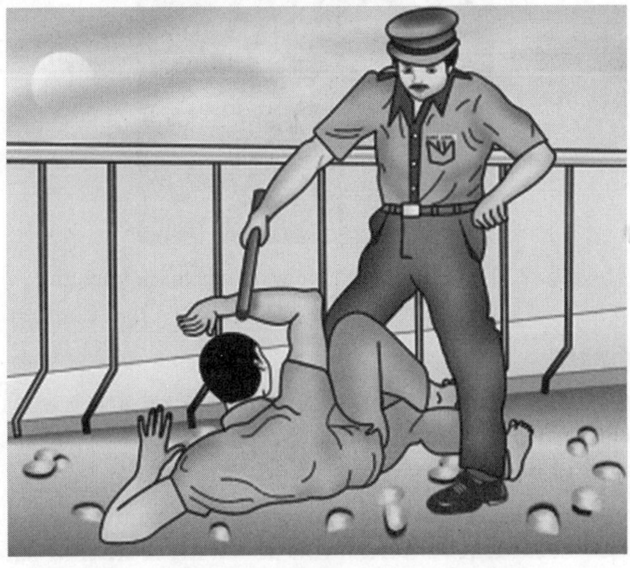

Fig. 2.17A: Mechanism of nightstick fracture

How does the patient present? Clinical Features

The patient presents with

- Pain,
- Swelling and
- Deformity along the subcutaneous border of the forearm.
- Rotational movements of the forearm are restricted.

Radiograph

The AP, lateral views of the forearm helps to make a diagnosis (Fig. 2.17B).

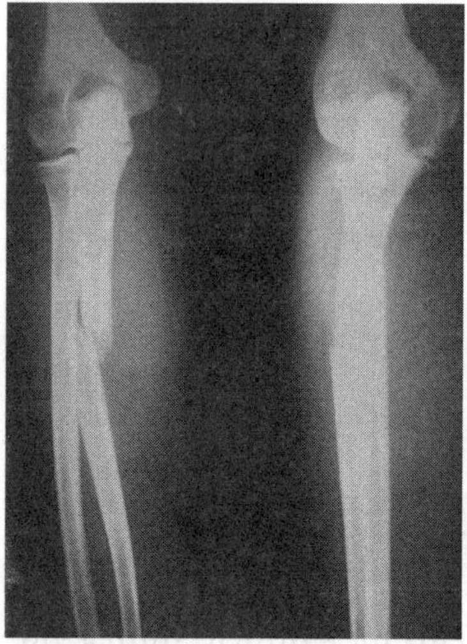

Fig. 2.17B: Radiograph showing nightstick fracture

Treatment

Conservative methods: The type I fractures are treated by immobilization with an above elbow plaster slab or cast for a period of 3–4 weeks.

Surgery: Type II and III varieties are treated by open reduction and rigid internal fixation with plate and screws.

DISTAL RADIUS FRACTURE

These are either extra-articular or intraarticular fractures and is classified based on the mechanism of injury.

Types: They are classified into five types namely:

Type I: Extra-articular metaphyseal fractures (e.g. Colles' fracture, Smith fracture). These are caused by bending forces.

Type II: Intra-articular fractures and include Barton both dorsal and volar and Radial styloid process fractures. They are caused by shearing forces.

Type III: Intra-articular fractures and metaphyseal impaction. Radial Pilon fractures fall in this group. They are caused by compression forces.

Type IV: These are avulsion radiocarpal injuries.

Type V: Multiple comminuted fractures and are due to high velocity forces.

Treatment Plan in a Nutshell

Type I: Colles or Smith' fractures can usually managed by closed reduction and plaster casting. Unstable fractures may require percutaneous fixation, plate and screws fixation and communited fractures need external fixators.

Type II: Usually, the Barton types require open reduction and rigid internal fixation (Ellis' plates).

Type III: Combination of open and closed techniques, wire fixation, open reduction and bone grafting after plating are some of the options.

Type IV: Avulsion fractures are treated by sutures, K-wire fixation, external fixation, etc.

Type V: Due to severe comminution open reduction is difficult. Fixation methods may require a combination of K-wire fixation and or external fixations.

WHAT IS NEW?

Distraction plate internal fixation: This is an alternative to external fixation and a distraction plate is used to provide internal distraction forces thereby eliminating the complications of external fixators.

COMMINUTED DISTAL RADIAL FRACTURE

Medoff developed both methods of percutaneous K-wire fixation and plates as when used alone either techniques were found wanting. He described five columns namely:

Radial column: Fixed with radial pin plate consisting of distal K-wire fixation and proximal screws through a radial buttress plate.

Dorsal cortical wall: Treated as dorsal Barton.

Dorsal ulnar split: Fixed with ulnar pin plate as described above. Wire form implants are used to stabilize the dorsal cortical wall.

Volar rim: Treatment as in volar barton with L-shaped buttress plate.

Central intraarticular fragments: Treatment is with the Trimed system.

DISTAL FOREARM FRACTURES

COLLES' FRACTURE

This is also called as **Poutteau's** fracture in many parts of the world. Abraham Colles first described it in the year 1814.

Definition

It is not just fracture lower end of radius but a fracture dislocation of the inferior radioulnar joint. The fracture occurs about 1½″ (about 2.5 cm) above the carpal extremity of the radius (Fig. 2.18).

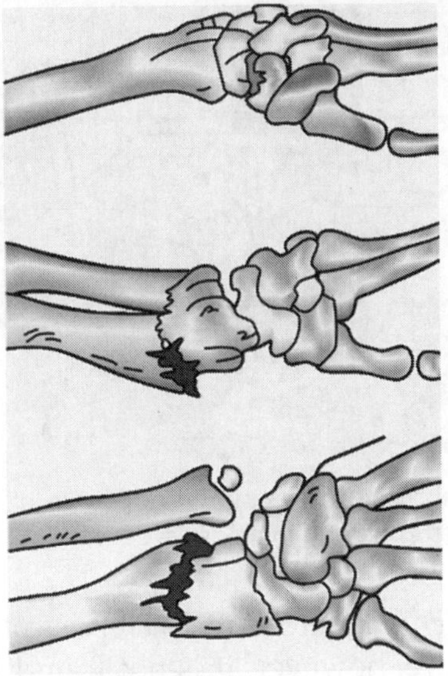

Fig. 2.18: Colles' fracture

Following this fracture, some deformity will remain throughout the life but pain decreases and movements increase gradually.

Mechanism of Injury

The common mode of injury is fall on an outstretched hand with dorsiflexion ranging from 40–90° (average 60°) (Fig. 2.19).

The force required to cause this fracture is 192 kg in women and 282 kg in men.

Fracture pattern: It is usually sharp on the palmar aspect and comminution on the dorsal surface of the lower end of radius.

How does the patient present? Clinical Features

- Usually, the patient is an elderly female in her 60s and the history given is a trivial fall on an outstretched hand.
- The patient complains of pain, swelling, deformity and other usual features of fracture at the lower end of radius.

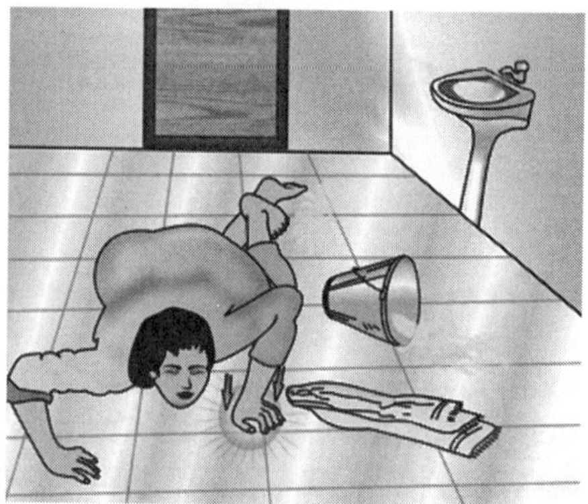

Fig. 2.19: Colles' fracture is usually due to a slip and fall on the outstretched hands in elderly females

- Though *dinner fork* deformity is a classical deformity in a Colles' fracture, however, it is not found in all cases but seen only if there is a dorsal tilt or rotation of the distal fragment (Figs 2.18 and 2.20).
- However, the styloid process test is more reliable.
- There are six classical displacements in a Colles' fracture.

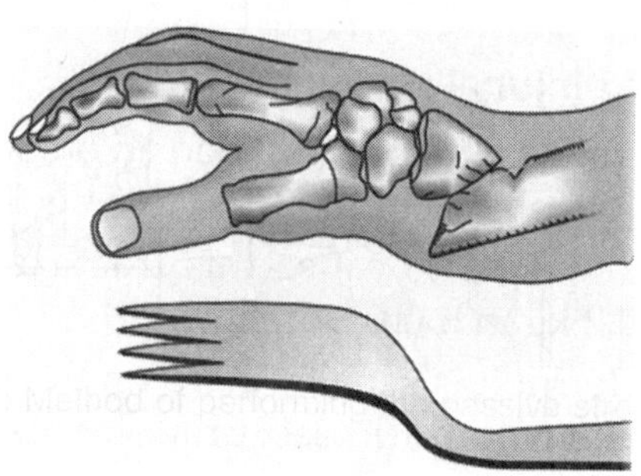

Fig. 2.20: Colles' fracture (A dinner fork deformity)

Did you know?

Dinner fork deformity is also called:

- Silver fork deformity.
- Spoon-shaped deformity.

Styloid Process Test

Normally, the radial styloid process is lower by 1.3 cm when compared to the ulnar styloid process. In Colles' both radial and ulnar styloid processes are at the same level and are found in all displacements of Colles' fracture. *Hence, this is a more reliable sign than dinner fork deformity* (Figs 2.21A and B).

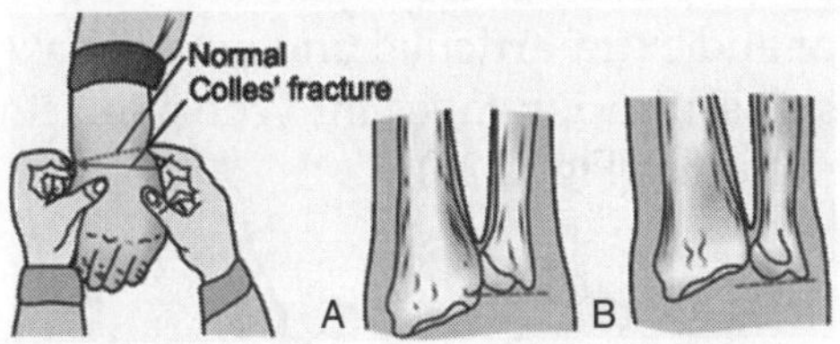

Figs 2.21A and B: Styloid process test: (A) Normal (B) In Colles' fractures

> *Note:* Dinner fork deformity is seen only in *d*orsal displacement and *D*orsal tilt in a Colles' fracture (note the *d's*).

Radiology

Radiographs of the wrist (Figs 2.22A and B) both AP and lateral views of the affected wrist and lower end of the radius are taken. The points noted in the AP view are metaphyseal comminution, fracture line extending into the radiocarpal or inferior radioulnar joint and fracture of the ulnar styloid process (seen in about 60% of the cases).

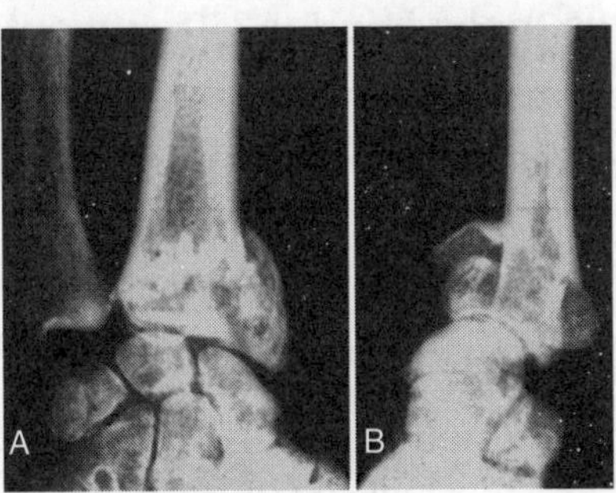

Figs 2.22 A and B: Radiographs showing Colles' fracture: (A) AP view, and (B) Lateral view

In the lateral view, the points noted are dorsal displacement and dorsal tilt of the distal fragment, sharp palmar surface and dorsal comminution of the lower end of radius, distal radioulnar joint subluxation, etc.

Classification

Contrary to popular belief, Colles' fracture is both intraarticular and extra-articular and not only extraarticular. Frykmann's classification takes into consideration both and the fracture of ulna (Fig. 2.23).

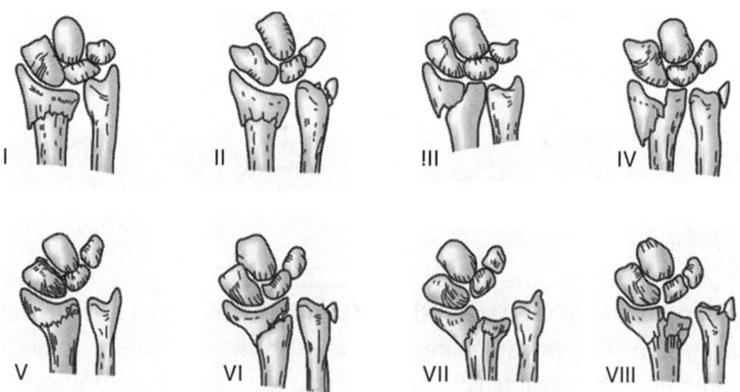

Fig. 2.23: Frykmann's varieties Colles' fracture

How to manage these injuries? Treatment Methods

Aim The aim of treatment is to restore fully functional hand with no residual deformity. The treatment methods include conservative methods, operative methods and external fixators (Figs 2.24 to 2.26).

Conservative Methods

Here fracture reduction is carried out by closed methods under general anesthesia (GA) or local anesthesia (LA). The examiner holds the hand of the patient as if to shake hand. With an assistant giving counteraction by holding the

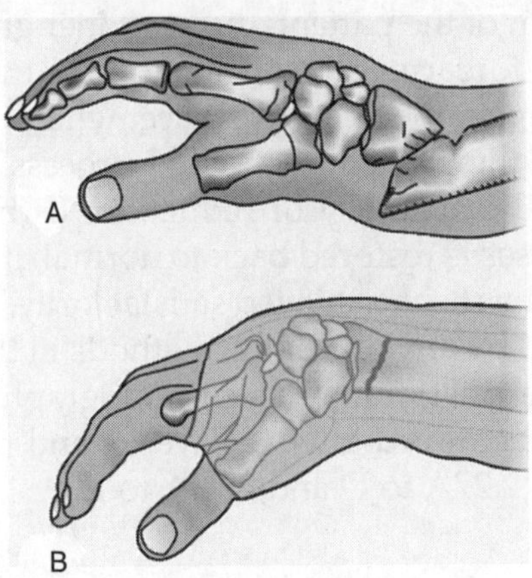

Figs 2.24A and B: (A) Atypical Colles' fracture, (B) Atypical Colles' cast

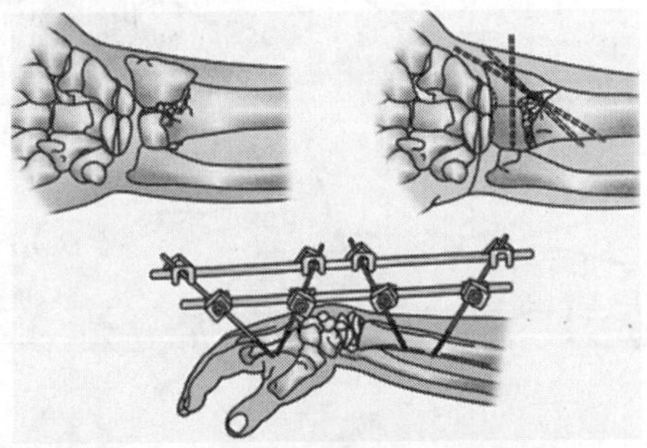

Fig. 2.25: Treatment method of Colles' fracture by external fixation

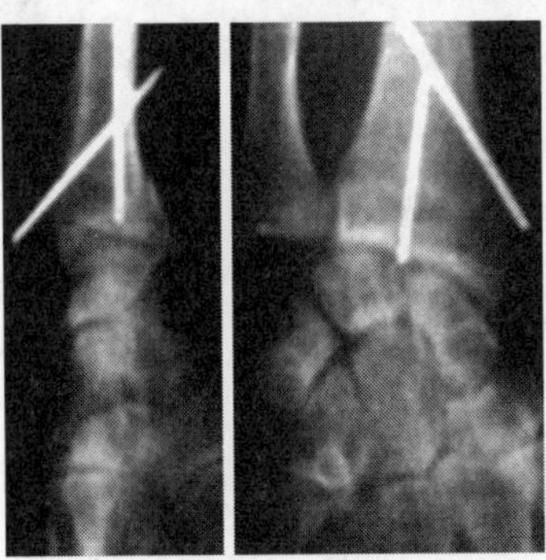

Fig. 2.26: Radiographs showing distal radius fracture percutaneous fixation

forearm or arm of the patient, the examiner gives traction in the line of the forearm. This disimpacts the fracture and the examiner corrects the other displacements of the fracture. At the end of the procedure, styloid process test is carried out to check the accuracy of reduction. If the level of the styloid processes is restored back to normal, it indicates that the reduction has been achieved satisfactorily. Then the limb is immobilized by any one of the methods in the table above (mainly Colles' cast) and a check radiograph is taken. The plaster cast is removed after 6–8 weeks and physiotherapy is begun (Figs 2.27A to D and 2.28A to I).

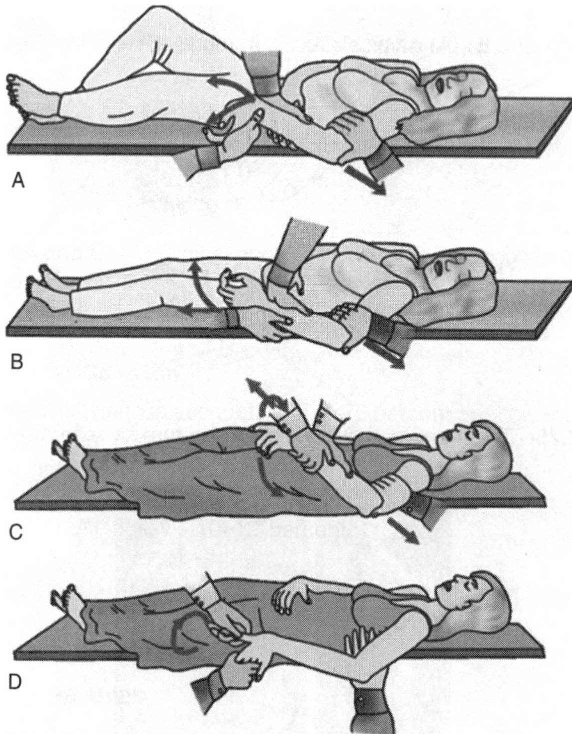

Figs 2.27A to D: Step-by-step closed reduction methods of Colles' fracture in an elderly woman: (A) Disimpaction, (B) Correcting anteroposterior displacements, (C) Correcting medial and lateral displacements, (D) Final manipulation

Colles' cast

It is a below elbow cast in supination and ideally, it has to meet the following four criteria:

- Firm fit at the dorsum.
- Firm fit at the volar fracture apex.
- Just snugly fitting at the forearm.
- Metacarpophalangeal joints should be free to move.

Technique of closed reduction and application of a colles' cast under local anesthesia (Figs 2.28A to I)

What is new?

Sonographically guided closed reduction is an accurate, radiation free, simple tool that is as accurate as the conventional radiographic techniques.

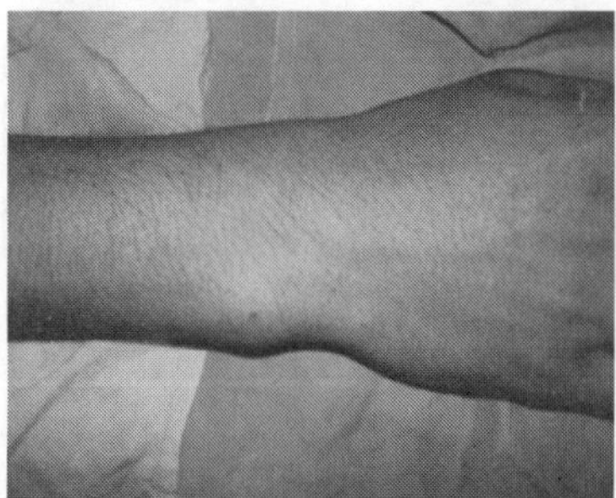

Fig. 2.28A: Dinner fork deformity

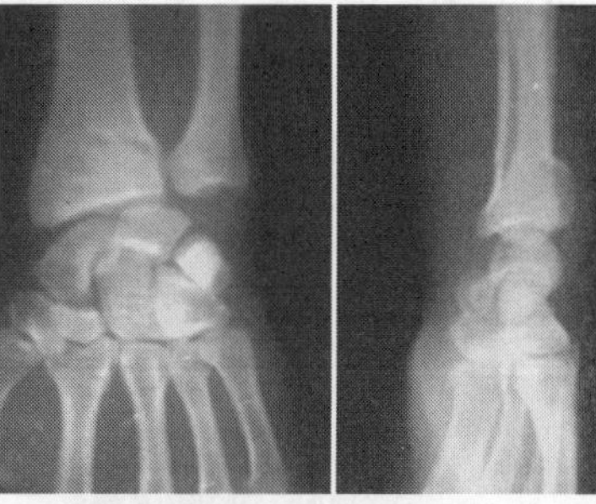

Fig. 2.28B: Radiograph showing AP and lateral views

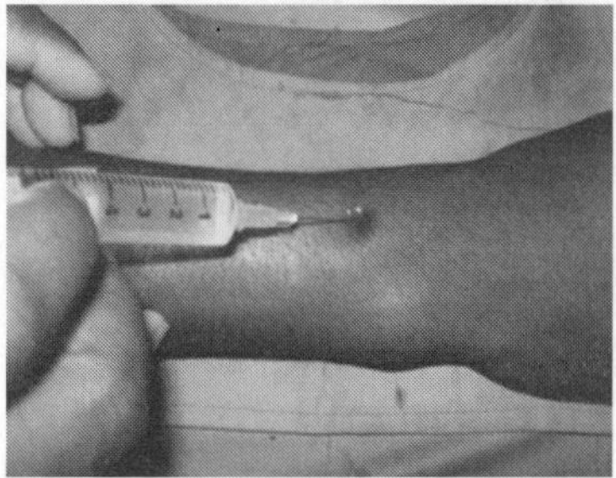

Fig. 2.28C: Injecting local anesthetic into the fracture site

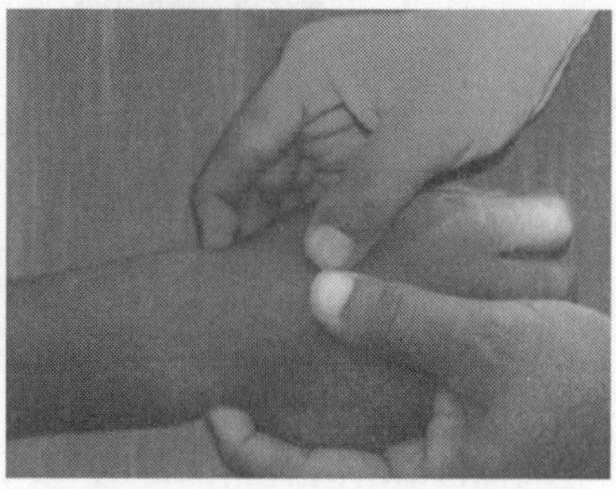

Fig. 2.28D: The styloid process test

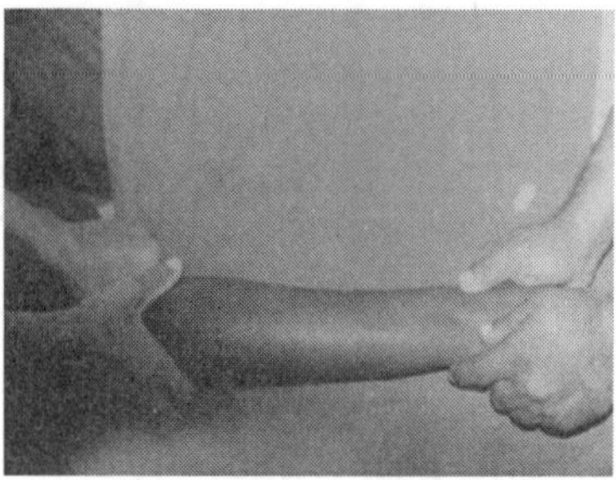

Fig. 2.28E: Reduction by traction and countertraction

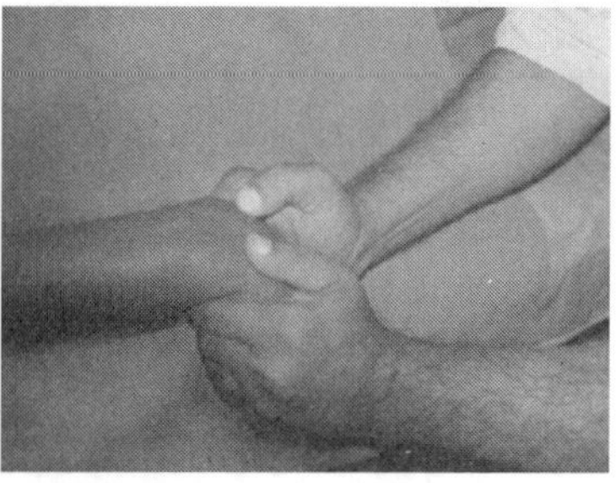

Fig. 2.28F: Manipulation of the fracture

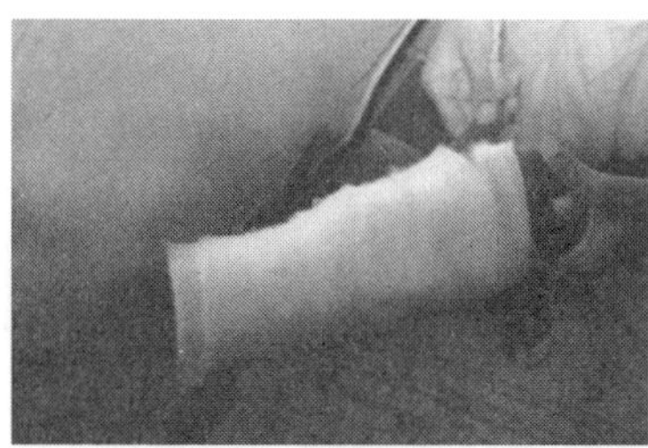

Fig. 2.28G: Application of soff ban

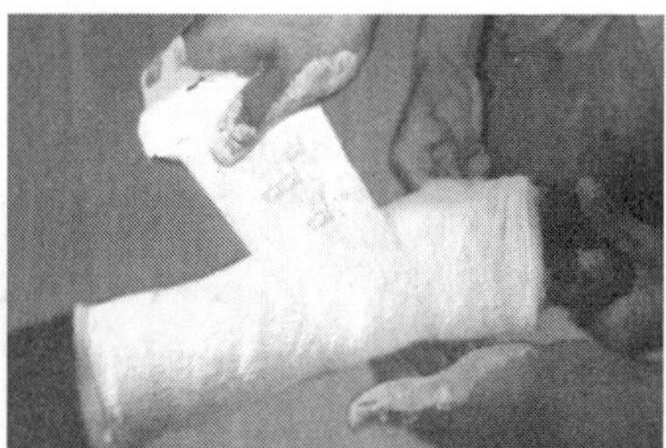

Fig. 2.28H: Application of the cast

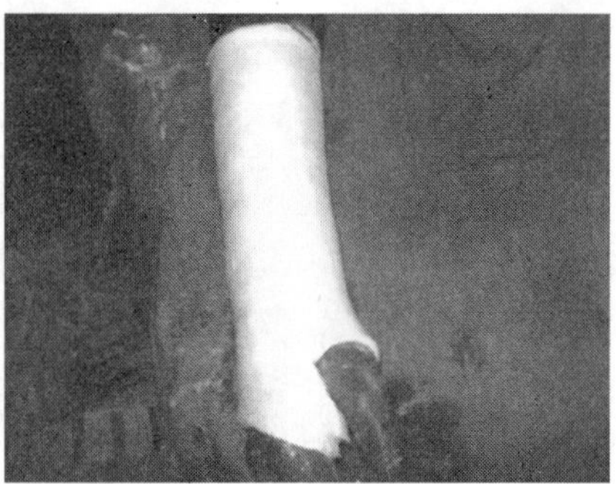

Fig. 2.28I: Colles' cast final presentation

The common causes for failure of reduction are incomplete reduction of the palmar fracture line and dorsal comminution of the lower end of radius.

Vital facts

Do you know the acceptable limits of Colles' fracture after reduction?

- A dorsal tilt of less than 10 degrees.
- A radial shortening of less than 5 mm.

Operative Methods

Operative treatment is rarely required for Colles' fracture and may be required in the following situations:

Indications: Extensive comminution, impaction, median nerve entrapment and associated injuries in adults.

Modalities of operative treatment: Depending upon the degree of comminution and the intraarticular extensions, one of the following surgical methods is chosen:

Closed reduction and percutaneous pinning with K-wires: Here, after closed reduction by the usual methods, the fracture fragments are held together by percutaneous pinning by one or two K-wires.

Arm control: This method is known to prevent collapse and gives good results in a few select cases.

Salient Features of Percutaneous Fixation

- It is becoming popular, as it is simple.
- It prevents redisplacement.
- Always needs an external support.
- One of the cortexes should not be comminuted.
- Preferably two pins are used (one radial and other dorsal).
- Care should be taken not to injure the radial sensory branch, the tendons, etc.

Open reduction in certain fractures involving the rim of the distal articular surfaces (Barton's variety), open reduction and plate fixation (Ellis' plate) is advocated (Fig. 2.30).

Indications: Same as for external fixation and for marginal volar or dorsal Barton's fractures.

Technique of closed reduction and percutaneous fixation with K-wires under GA (Figs 2.29A to P)

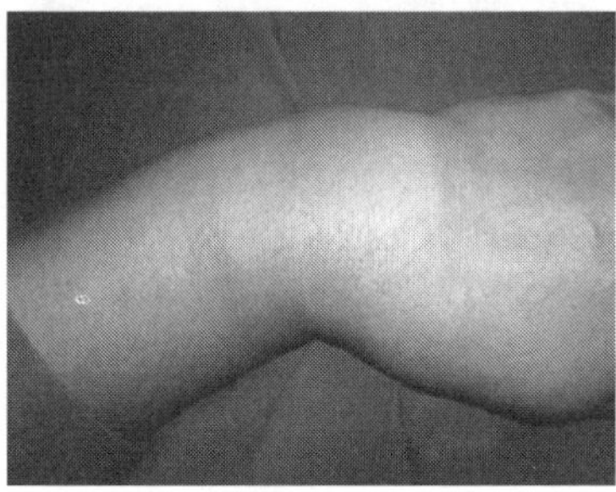

Fig. 2.29A: Gross deformity as viewed from the radial side

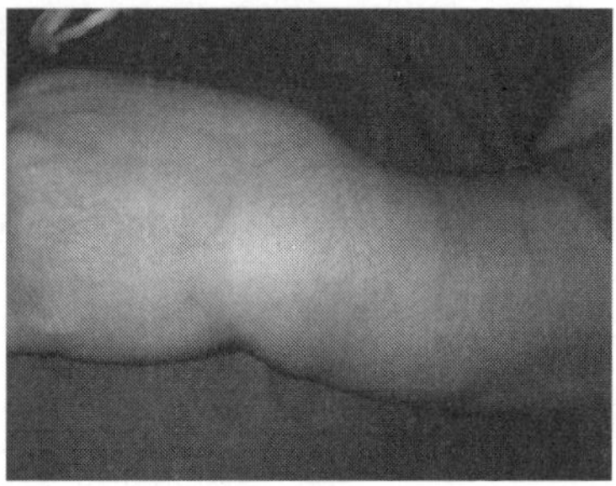

Fig. 2.29B: Deformity as viewed from the ulnar side

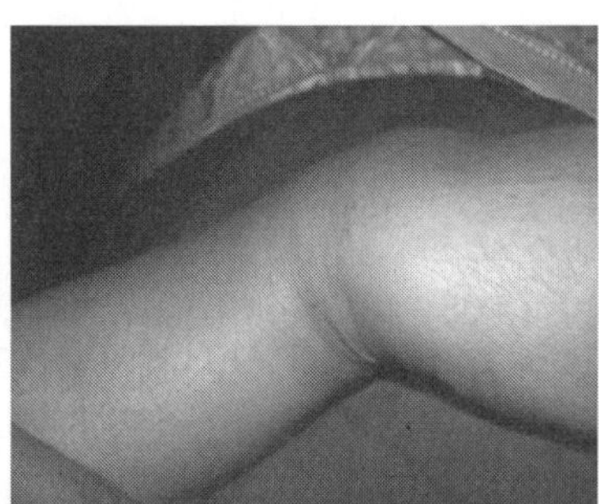

Fig. 2.29C: Deformity as viewed from the sides

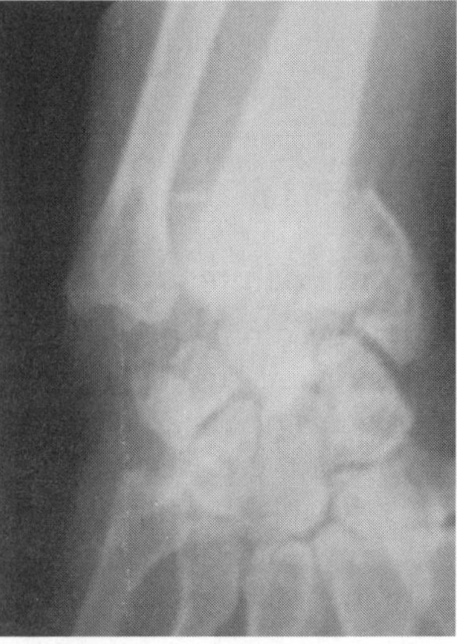

Fig. 2.29D: Radiograph showing communited intraarticular fracture of radius and subluxation of INFRUD

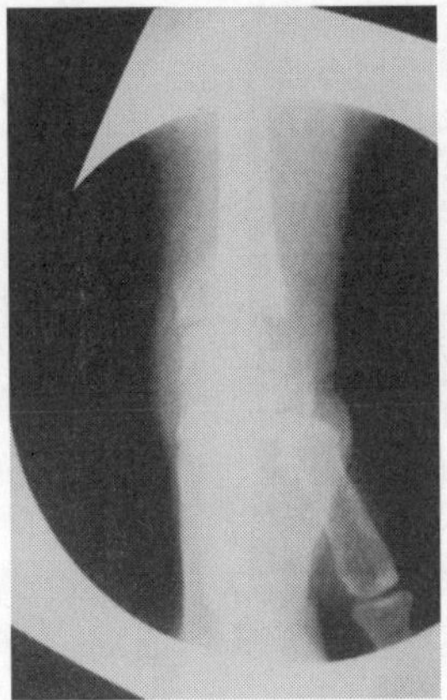

Fig. 2.29E: Radiograph showing lateral view

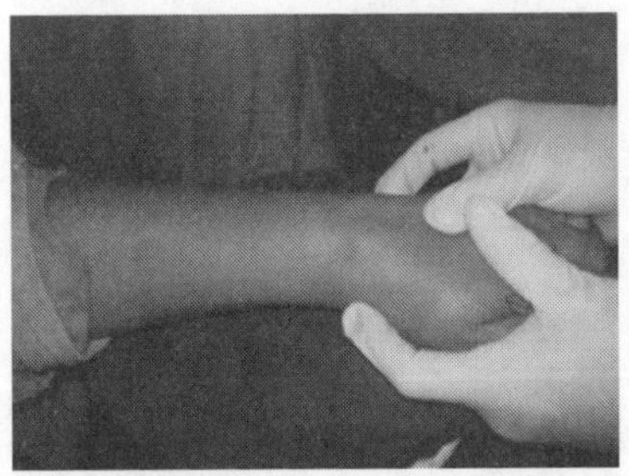

Fig. 2.29F: The styloid process test before closed reduction

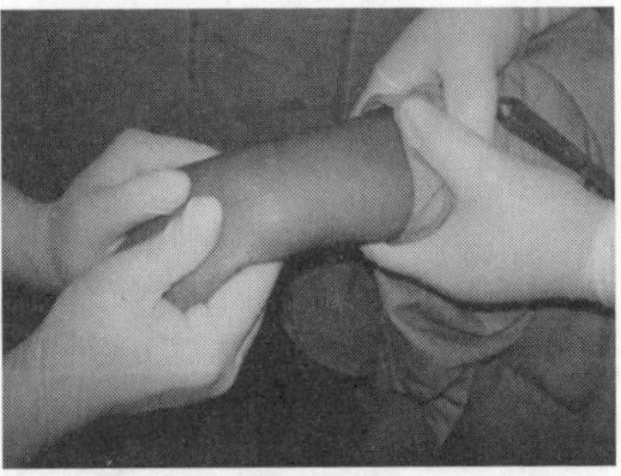

Fig. 2.29G: Reduction by traction and counter traction

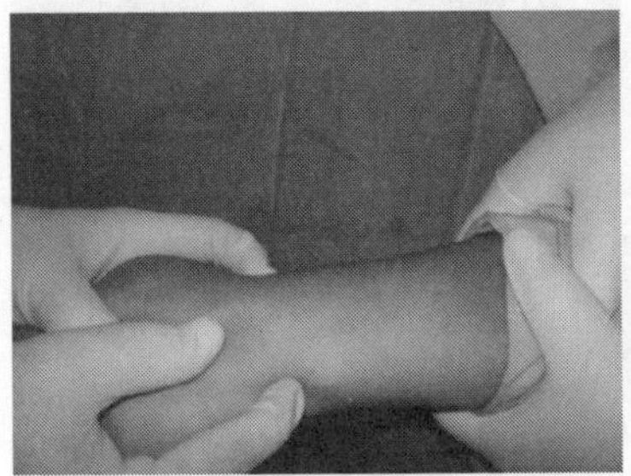

Fig. 2.29H: Checking for the satisfactory reduction

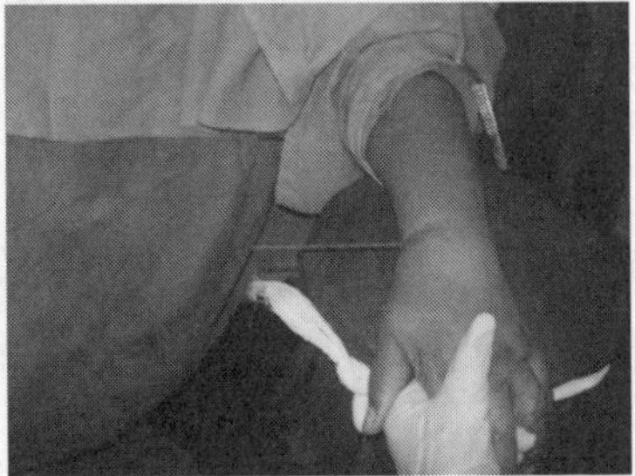

Fig. 2.29I: Percutaneous K-wire fixation

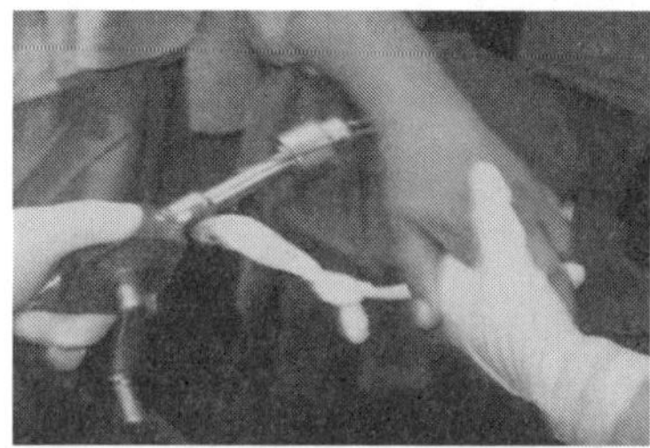

Fig. 2.29J: Placement of second pin

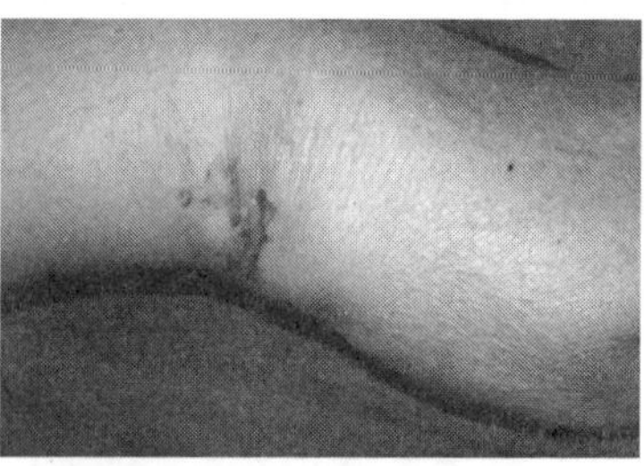

Fig. 2.29K: Pins cut flush to the skin

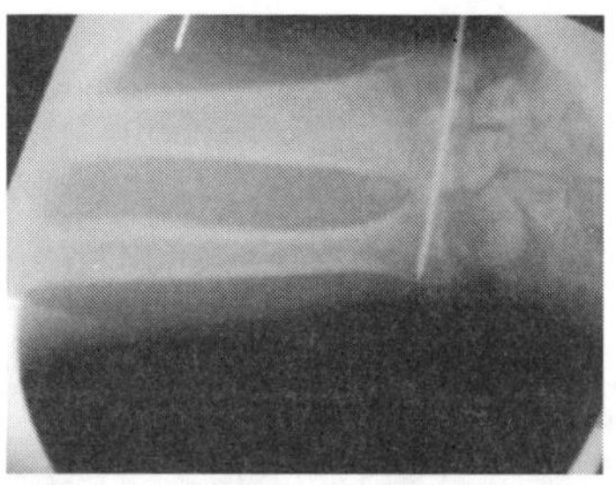

Fig. 2.29L: C-arm view after the first pin

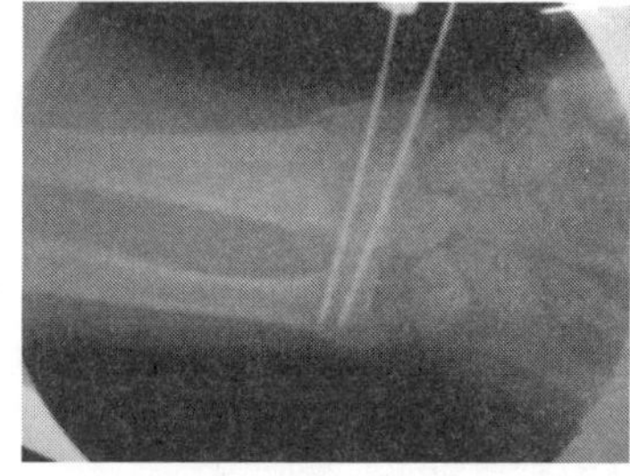

Fig. 2.29M: C-arm view after the second pin

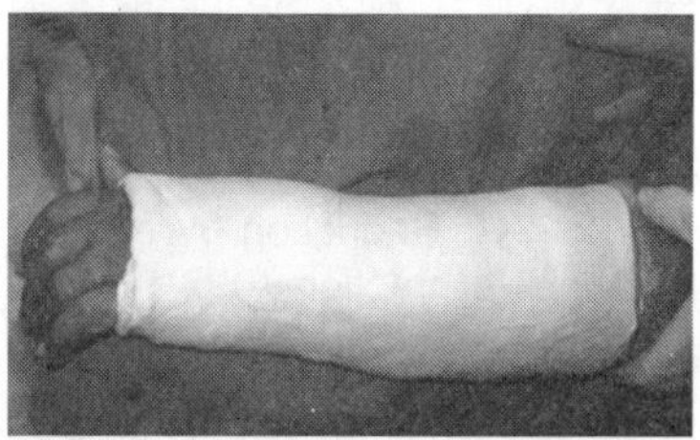

Fig. 2.29N: Colles' cast applied

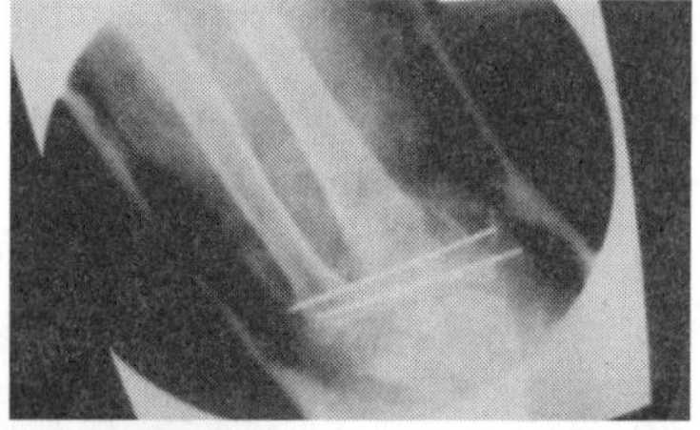

Fig. 2.29O: C-arm view after the pins and plaster

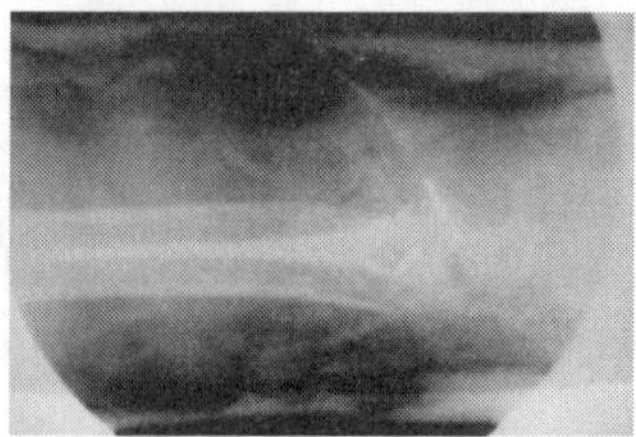

Fig. 2.29P: Lateral view

Advantages

- Provides buttress
- Resists compression
- Load sharing
- Early mobilization.

What is new? Arthroscopically assisted internal fixation

External fixators (Fig. 2.30): These are found to be extremely useful in highly comminuted fractures, unstable fractures, compound fractures and bilateral Colles' fracture. Through a lightweight UMEX frames, two pins are placed in the forearm bones and two pins in the metacarpal bones of the hand. These pins are then fixed to an external frame and the fracture fragments are held in position by ligamentotaxis. The frame should be applied after obtaining closed reduction by the usual method.

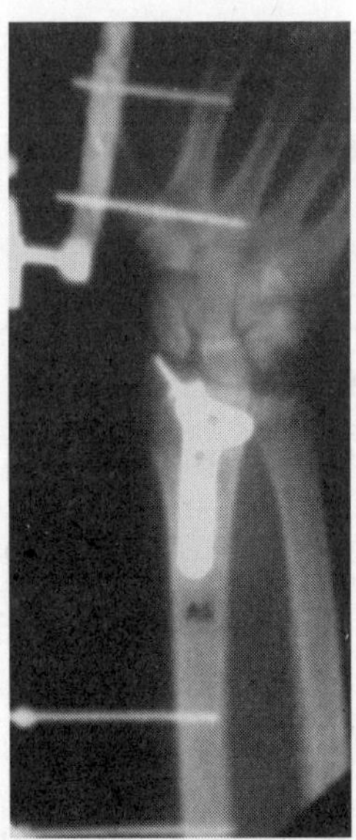

Fig. 2.30: Radiograph showing distal radius fracture being treated by both external fixator and plate screws

What is new?

Closed reduction and finger-trap traction is found to ensure better reduction and a lower rate of redisplacement than just manual manipulation (Fig. 2.31).

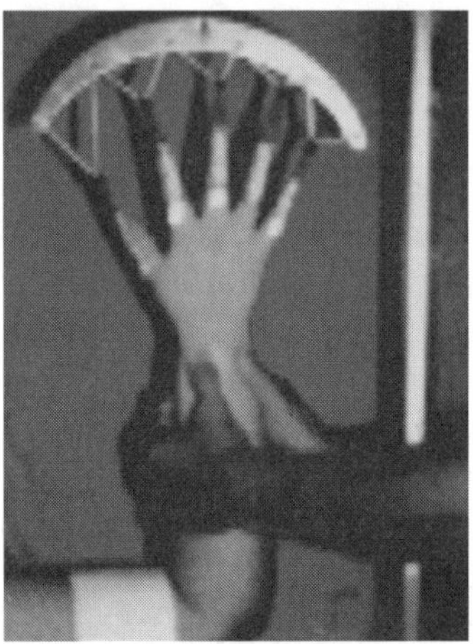

Fig. 2.31: Finger-trap traction for fracture reduction

What are the problems or complications

Few significant complications of Colles' fracture are discussed here.

Malunion This is the most common complication of Colles' fracture. Six important causes are responsible for it.

- *Improper reduction:* If the fracture is not reduced properly, in the initial stages it may result in malunion later.
- *Improper and inadequate immobilization:* This fracture needs to be immobilized at least for a period of six weeks failing which malunion results.
- *Comminuted dorsal surface:* Due to extensive comminution, the fracture collapses and recurs after reduction and casting.
- Osteoporosis may lead to collapse and recurrence.

- *Recurrence:* This is due to extensive comminution and osteoporosis.
- *Rupture of the distal radioulnar ligament:* This usually goes undetected in the initial stages of treatment and is responsible for the later recurrence.

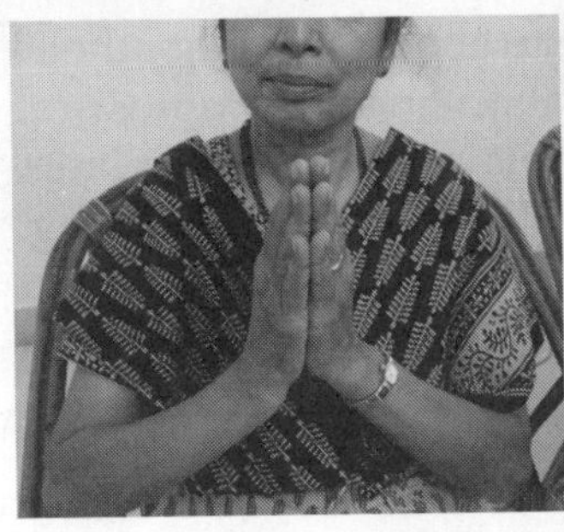
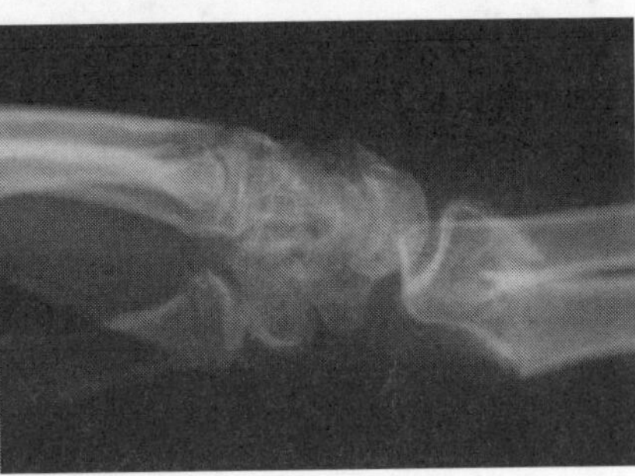

Fig. 2.32

Treatment

There are six options of treatment in a malunited Colles' fracture

- No treatment is required if the patient has no functional abnormality.
- Remanipulation is attempted if fracture is less than 2 weeks old.
- Darrach's operation is more often indicated if the patient complains of functional disability.
- Corrective osteotomy and grafting if the patient wants cosmetic correction and if the patient is young (Fernandez and Campbell).

  Fernandez is a dorsal wedge osteotomy and Campbell is a lateral wedge osteotomy.
- *Arthrodesis (for intraarticular fracture):* The patient complains of pain in the wrist joint due to traumatic osteoarthritis following an intraarticular fracture. In these patients, arthrodesis of the wrist in functional position is the surgery of choice.

- Combination of these like Darrach's operation with osteotomy, etc. is also tried in some situations.

Rupture of extensor pollicis tendon: This occurs due to the attrition of the tendon as it glides over the sharp fracture surfaces. This usually occurs after 4–6 weeks and may be repaired or left alone with no residual disability.

Sudeck's osteodystrophy: This is due to abnormal sympathetic response, which causes vasodilatation and osteoporosis at the fracture site. The patient complains of pain, swelling, painful wrist movements and red-stretched shiny skin (Fig. 2.33). Treatment consists of immobilization of the affected part with plaster splints, injection of local anesthetics near the sympathetic ganglion in the axilla or cervical sympathectomy in extreme cases.

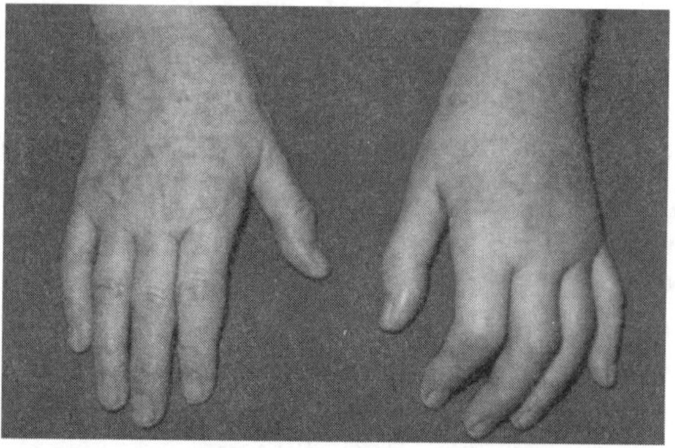

Fig. 2.33: Sudeck's osteodystrophy (Clinical photo)

Frozen hand shoulder syndrome: This is a troublesome complication, which develops due to unnecessary voluntary shoulder immobilization by the patient on the affected side for fear of fracture displacements. It is said that the patient has performed a *mental amputation* and kept the limb still (Fig. 2.34).

Carpal tunnel syndrome: Malunion of Colles' fracture crowds the carpal tunnel and compresses the median nerve.

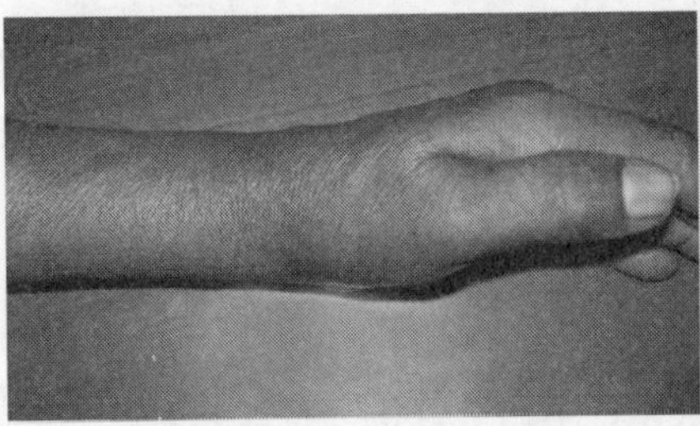
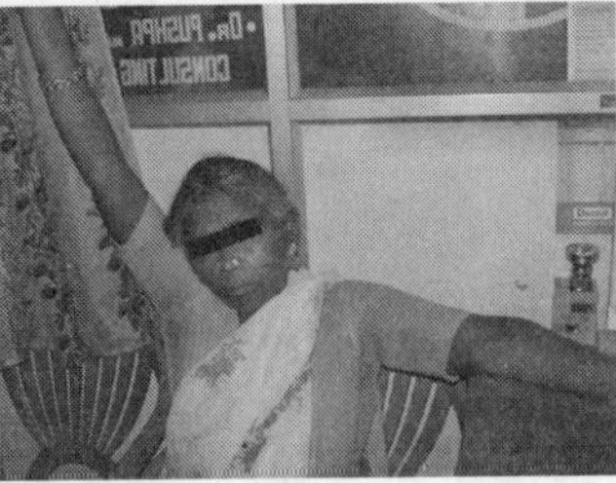

Fig. 2.34: Clinical photo showing frozen hand shoulder syndrome

Nonunion: This is extremely rare in Colles' fracture because of the cancellous nature of the bone, which enables the fracture to unite well. However, soft tissue interposition may cause this problem. The treatment consists of open reduction, rigid internal fixation and bone grafting.

Quick facts

Colles' fracture—why is it called fracture of 6?

- Common at 60 years.
- Force required to cause Colles' fracture are multiples of 6.
- 6 classical displacements.
- 6 methods of fracture immobilization.
- 6 weeks immobilization.
- 6 important early and late complications.
- 6 causes for malunion.
- 6 methods of managing malunion.
- 60 percent cases have fracture ulnar styloid.

GALEAZZI'S FRACTURE

Introduction

This is a fracture of radius at the junction of middle and distal third with associated subluxation or dislocation of the distal radioulnar joint. Subluxation of this joint may be present initially or occur during treatment (Figs 2.35A and B).

French people call this fracture *reverse Monteggia.*

Campbell called it as *fracture of necessity* since it always requires open reduction and internal fixation (ORIF).

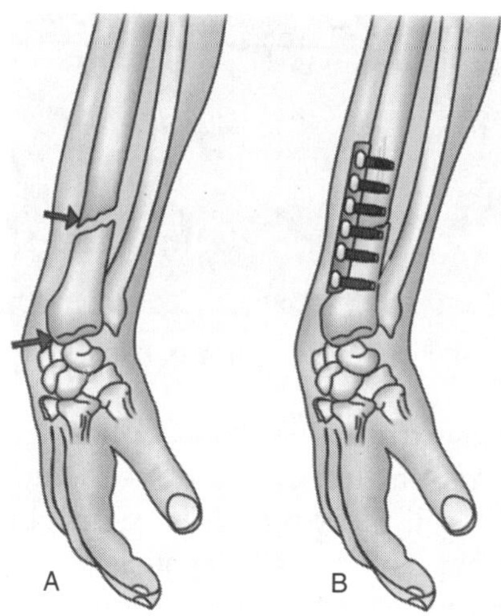

Figs 2.35A and B: (A) Galeazzi's fracture, and (B) ORIF with DCP plate and screws (Preferred method)

The following are the major deforming forces causing loss of reduction and difficulty in reduction (Fig. 2.36).

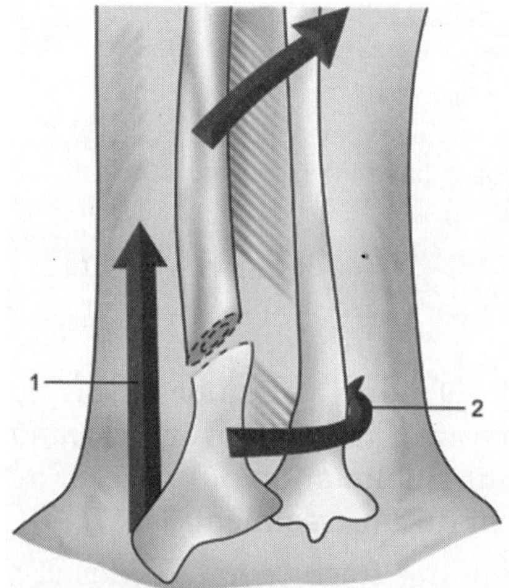

Fig. 2.36: Displacing forces in Galeazzi's fractures, (1) Brachioradialis, and (2) Pronator quadratus

- Gravity acting through the hand.
- Insertion of pronator quadratus pulls the distal fragment in proximal and volar direction.
- Brachioradialis uses the distal radioulnar joint as a pivot and causes shortening.
- Abductors and extensors of the thumb cause shortening and relaxation of the radiocarpal ligament.

Incidence: It is three times as common as Monteggia's fracture.

Mechanism of Injury

- Fall on an outstretched hand with marked pronation of the forearm.
- Direct blow on the dorsolateral side of the forearm.

How does the patient present? Clinical Features

The patient complains of pain, swelling and deformity of the lower end of the forearm. Pronation and supination are severely restricted. All other features of fractures are present.

Radiograph

Important radiological features of Galleazzi's fracture are as shown in the box (Fig. 2.37A).

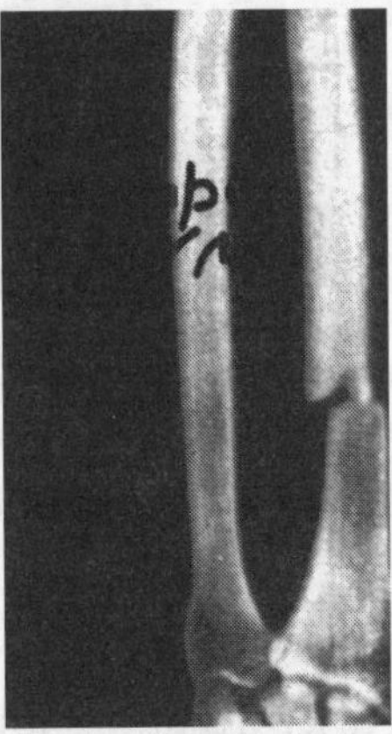

Fig. 2.37A: Radiograph showing Galeazzi's fracture

AP view	Lateral view
• Fracture radius, transverse or short oblique • Comminution is less • Distal radioulnar joint is dislocated • Radius appears short	• Radius is angulated dorsally • Head of the ulna is prominent dorsally

How to manage these injuries? Treatment

Closed reduction is usually not successful due to the deforming forces of the muscles. Hence, ORIF is the preferred method of treatment (Fig 2.37B). Intramedullary nails and small plates do not provide adequate fixation, long plate (LCDCP plate) and screws are thus used and the dislocated distal radioulnar joint may be fixed with K-wire.

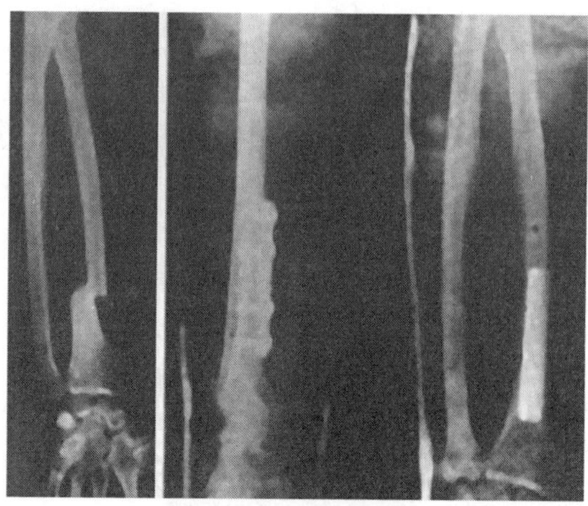

Fig. 2.37B: Radiograph showing Galeazzi's fracture fixation

What are the problems? Complications

- Nonunion and
- Malunion are notorious complications.
- Angulation of the fracture and subluxation of the distal radioulnar joint can also occur. Rarely entrapment of

extensor carpi ulnaris tendon in distal radioulnar joint is encountered.

ESSEX-LOPRESTI FRACTURE

Introduction

This is a fracture of the radial head with injury to the distal radioulnar joint and tearing of the interosseous membrane proximally.

Mechanism of Injury

A heavy fall on the outstretched hands.

How does the patient present? Clinical Features

- Pain and swelling in the radial head region.
- Pain in the region of the distal radioulnar joint should alert of a possibility.
- Pain in the wrist could be due to ulnar carpal impingement and pain in the elbow could be due to radiocapitellar impingement.

Radiograph

It is a relatively rare fracture and in order to avoid missing it, radiograph of the forearm and wrist joint should be taken in all cases of fracture of head of the radius.

How to manage these fractures? Treatment

Open reduction and internal fixation of the proximal radial fracture and pinning of the inferior radioulnar joint is the treatment method of choice.

If there is disruption of distal radioulnar joint and if the radial head fracture is grossly comminuted then, excision head of the radius is done. This is likely to aggravate the proximal migration of the radius. Hence, if fracture radial head needs excision, it has to be replaced by silastic prosthesis.

RADIAL STYLOID FRACTURE (Chauffeurs Fracture)

Introduction

Radial styloid fracture (Hutchinson's fracture) is similar to the posterior marginal fracture of the radius.

Mechanism

It is usually because of the starting crank of an engine being suddenly reversed by a backfire and striking the wrist with a force. It is common in chauffeurs and is an avulsion fracture of the radiocarpal ligament (Fig. 2.38A).

> *Note:* These are also seen in motorcycle accidents and fall from heights.

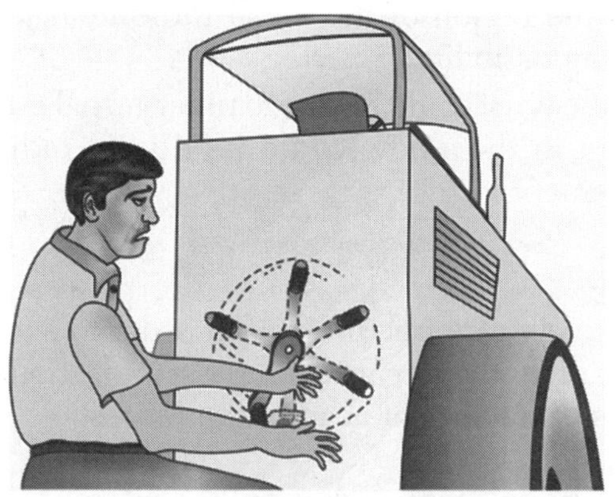

Fig. 2.38A: Mechanism of injury of Hutchinson's fracture

How does the patient present? Clinical Features

The patient complains of

- Pain,
- Swelling and
- Tenderness over the radial styloid process.
- Movement of the wrist, especially radial deviation, is painful.

Radiographs

Radiograph AP view of the wrist shows it as a transverse fracture (Fig. 2.38B).

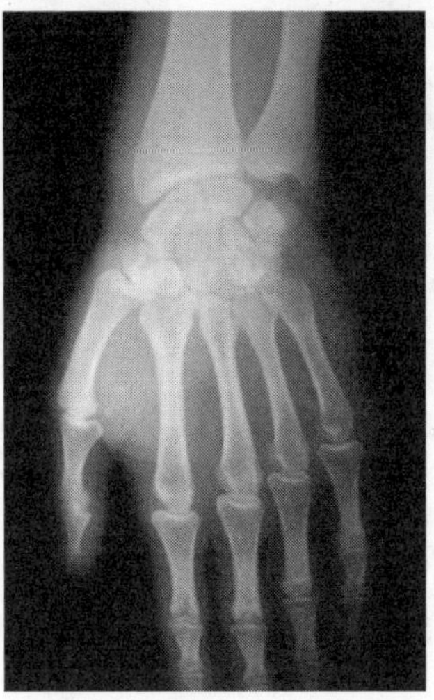

Fig. 2.38B: Radiograph showing radial styloid process fracture

How to manage this fracture? Treatment

This fracture is best treated by an above or below plaster slab or cast in undisplaced fractures and closed reduction and above elbow plaster cast if it is displaced. However, unstable fractures need percutaneous fixation with K-wire.

SMITH'S FRACTURE

Introduction

It is a fracture of distal one-third of radius with palmar displacement. Hence, it is called as *reverse Colles' fracture*.

However, it is less common than Colles' it is readily confused with Colles' fracture.

It has a clear fracture dorsally with comminution of the palmar surface (Figs 2.39A and B).

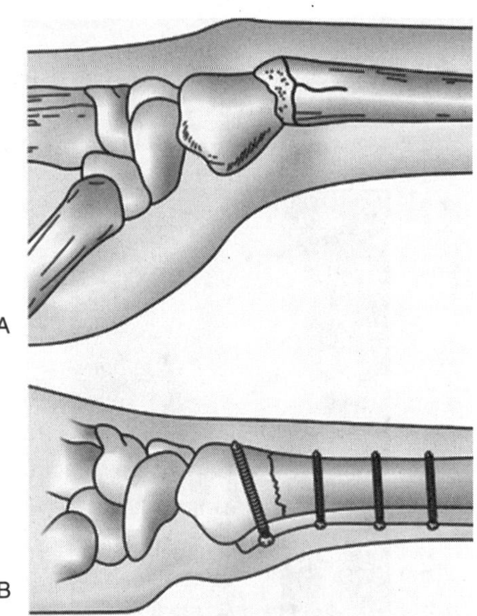

Figs 2.39A and B: (A) Smith's fracture, and (B) Method of fixation of Smith's fracture

Did you know?

Smith's fracture occurs about 1/10 as frequent as Colles' fracture. The greatest problem with this fracture is executing the treatment mistaking it to be a Colles' fracture!

Mechanism of Injury

There are three modes of injury like fall on the back of the dorsum of the hand, fall on the forearm in supination and a direct blow to the flexed hand.

How does the patient present? Clinical Features

The patient complains of

- Pain,
- Swelling
- Tenderness
- Deformity

- Loss of wrist functions.
- The deformity is opposite to that of Colles' fracture and is called the 'garden spade' deformity.

Radiograph

Anteroposterior view of the wrist shows the carpus proximally displaced. There will be anterior displacement of the fragment with palmar angulation of distal radial articular surface (Fig. 2.39C). The ulnar styloid process is frequently fractured.

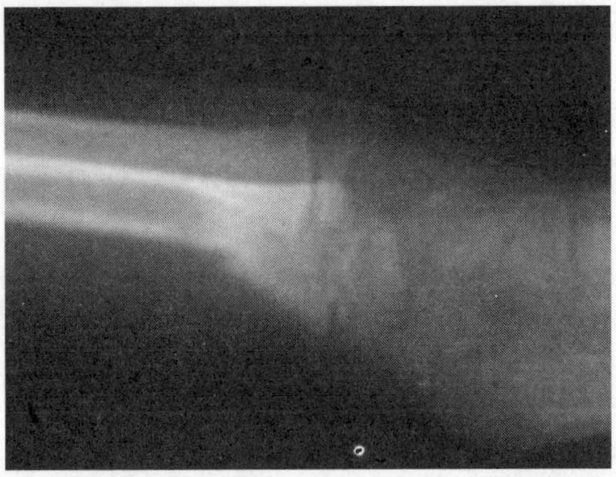

Fig. 2.39C: Radiograph showing Smith's fracture

How to manage these fractures? Treatment

Conservative methods: The treatment of choice is closed reduction and immobilization in a long arm cast with forearm in supination and wrist in extension.

Surgery: For unstable fractures, fixation with percutaneous K-wire or open reduction and plate fixation may be required (Fig. 2.39B).

Complications

- Misinterpretation of radiographs for Colles'.
- Other complication of Colles'.

BARTON'S FRACTURE

Introduction

Rim fractures of the distal radius are called Barton's fracture. Dorsal or volar rim could be involved and these fractures are invariably intraarticular.

DORSAL BARTON FRACTURE

Dorsal Barton is a dorsal rim fracture of distal radius with dorsal subluxation or dislocation. It is a variant of Colles' fracture (Fig. 2.40).

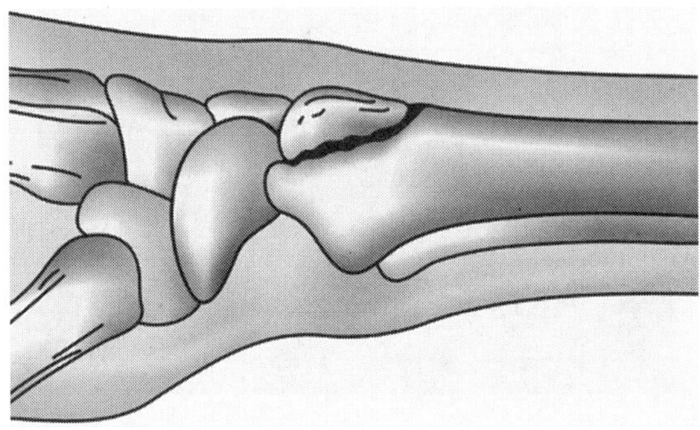

Fig. 2.40: Dorsal Barton's fracture

Mechanism

Fall with dorsiflexion and pronation of the distal forearm on a flexed wrist.

How does the patient present? Clinical Features

Patient complains of

- Severe pain
- Swelling
- Tenderness over the dorsum of the wrist and
- Restricted wrist movements with painful dorsiflexion.

Radiograph

Best seen on the lateral view. Dorsal lip of distal radial articular surface is displaced proximally and posteriorly and may be associated with dorsal subluxation of the wrist (Figs 2.41A and B).

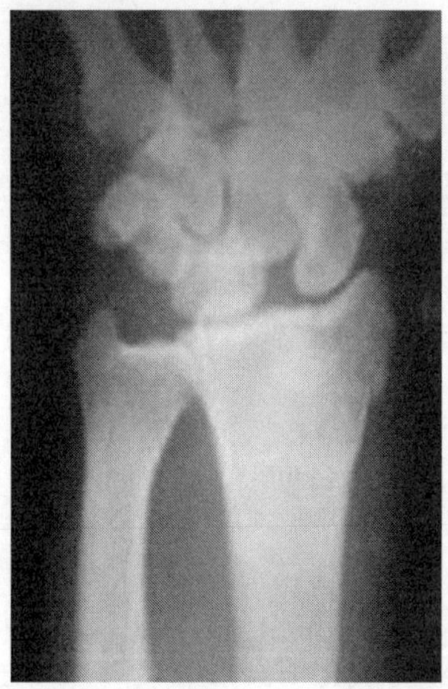

Fig. 2.41A: Radiograph showing dorsal Barton's fracture (AP view)

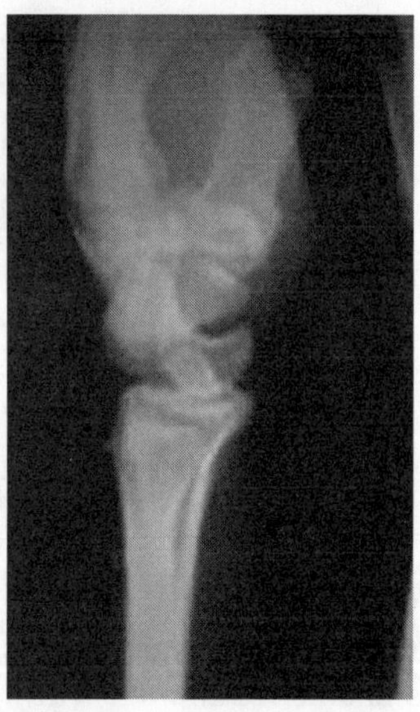

Fig. 2.41B: Radiograph showing dorsal Barton's fracture (lateral view)

How to manage these fractures? Treatment

Conservative Methods

Short arm plaster cast with the wrist joint in neutral position.

Surgery

- Unstable fracture is fixed by percutaneous pins or small screws.
- Open Reduction + Internal fixation with small plate and screws can be done but due to the extensor tendons may not be good option.

VOLAR BARTON FRACTURE (Palmar rim dislocation)

Volar Barton (Palmar rim dislocation) is a palmar rim fracture of distal radius (Fig. 2.42).

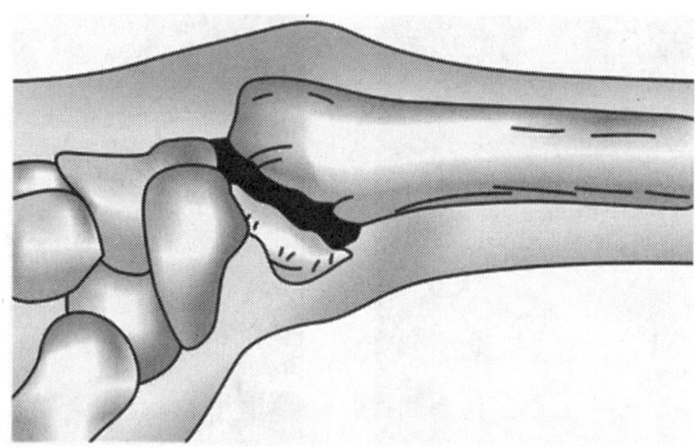

Fig. 2.42: Volar Barton's fracture

Mechanism

It is due to palmar tensile stress and dorsal shear stress and is usually combined with radial styloid fracture.

How does the patient present? Clinical Features

It consists of

- Pain
- Swelling
- Tenderness over the palmar surface of the wrist
- Loss of wrist movements.
- Palmar flexion is grossly restricted and painful.

Radiograph

Palmar rim of distal radial articular surface is displaced dorsally.

Proximally and posteriorly and may be associated with dorsal subluxation of the wrist (Fig. 2.43A).

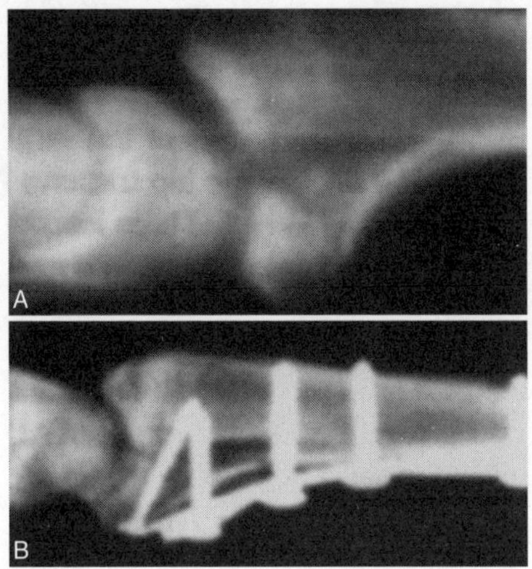

Figs 2.43A and B: Radiographs showing Volar Barton's fracture (A), fixed with plate and screws (B)

How to manage these injuries? Treatment Methods

Conservative

Reduction is simple, but retention is difficult. Long arm plaster cast is used for immobilization.

Surgery

If reduction does not remain satisfactorily with wrist in neutral or slight palmar flexion, fixation with K-wire, external fixators and buttress plate, etc. may be done.

Ellis T-shaped buttress plate fixation is the preferred method of treatment (Fig. 2.43B).

Index

Clinical Notes

Clinical Notes

Clinical Notes

Clinical Notes

Clinical Notes

Clinical Notes